# Frontiers in Anatomy

## *(Volume 1)*

### *Anatomy for Oral and Maxillofacial Radiology*

**Authored by**

**Plauto C. A. Watanabe**

*School of Dentistry of Ribeirão Preto, University of São Paulo, São Paulo, Brazil*

**Emiko S. Arita**

*School of Dentistry of University of São Paulo, São Paulo, Brazil*

**Angela J. Camargo**

*School of Dentistry of Ribeirão Preto, University of São Paulo, São Paulo, Brazil*

**&**

**Marina G. Baladi**

*School of Dentistry of University of São Paulo, São Paulo, Brazil*

## General:

1. Any dispute or claim arising out of or in connection with this License Agreement or the Work (including non-contractual disputes or claims) will be governed by and construed in accordance with the laws of the U.A.E. as applied in the Emirate of Dubai. Each party agrees that the courts of the Emirate of Dubai shall have exclusive jurisdiction to settle any dispute or claim arising out of or in connection with this License Agreement or the Work (including non-contractual disputes or claims).
2. Your rights under this License Agreement will automatically terminate without notice and without the need for a court order if at any point you breach any terms of this License Agreement. In no event will any delay or failure by Bentham Science Publishers in enforcing your compliance with this License Agreement constitute a waiver of any of its rights.
3. You acknowledge that you have read this License Agreement, and agree to be bound by its terms and conditions. To the extent that any other terms and conditions presented on any website of Bentham Science Publishers conflict with, or are inconsistent with, the terms and conditions set out in this License Agreement, you acknowledge that the terms and conditions set out in this License Agreement shall prevail.

**Bentham Science Publishers Ltd.**
Executive Suite Y - 2
PO Box 7917, Saif Zone
Sharjah, U.A.E.
Email: subscriptions@benthamscience.org

BENTHAM
SCIENCE

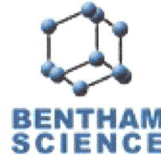

# CONTENTS

FOREWORD .......................................................................................................... i

PREFACE ............................................................................................................. ii

LIST OF CONTRIBUTORS ................................................................................. iii

CHAPTER 1 BASIC ASPECTS OF DENTAL RADIOGRAPHIC IMAGES ................. 1
*Plauto C. A. Watanabe, Emiko S. Arita, Angela J. Camargo* and *Marina G. Baladi*
INTRODUCTION [1] ........................................................................................... 1
IDEAL RADIOGRAPH ....................................................................................... 2
CONCLUSION .................................................................................................... 4
CONSENT FOR PUBLICATION ......................................................................... 4
CONFLICT OF INTEREST ................................................................................. 4
ACKNOWLEDGEMENTS ................................................................................... 4
REFERENCE ...................................................................................................... 4

CHAPTER 2 DENTAL RADIOGRAPHIC TECHNIQUES ...................................... 5
*Plauto C. A. Watanabe, Emiko S. Arita, Angela J. Camargo* and *Marina G. Baladi*
INTRAORAL EXAMINATIONS [1 - 3] ............................................................... 5
    Periapical Radiography ................................................................................... 5
    Interproximal Radiography (Bite-wing) ........................................................... 6
    Occlusal Radiography ..................................................................................... 7
EXTRAORAL EXAMINATIONS [1 - 3] .............................................................. 8
    Panoramic Radiography ................................................................................. 8
    Temporomandibular Joint Radiography (Transcranial) ..................................... 9
    Cephalometric Radiography ........................................................................... 9
    Teleradiograph (Lateral) ................................................................................ 9
    PA Skull ........................................................................................................ 10
    PA Projection (Waters) .................................................................................. 10
    Axial (Hirtz Projection) .................................................................................. 11
CONCLUSION .................................................................................................... 11
CONSENT FOR PUBLICATION ......................................................................... 12
CONFLICT OF INTEREST ................................................................................. 12
ACKNOWLEDGEMENTS ................................................................................... 12
REFERENCES .................................................................................................... 12

CHAPTER 3 ANATOMY OF INTRAORAL TECHNIQUES ................................... 13
*Plauto C. A. Watanabe, Emiko S. Arita, Angela J. Camargo* and *Marina G. Baladi*
PERIAPICAL AND INTERPROXIMAL RADIOGRAPHS [1 - 5] ........................... 13
    Dental Regions ............................................................................................... 13
    Central Region of Maxilla [1 - 5] .................................................................... 21
    Lateral Incisor and Canine Region (Fig. 21) [3 - 5] .......................................... 24
    Premolar and Molar Region [2 - 5] ................................................................. 27
    Molar Region [1 - 5] (Figs. 32-35) .................................................................. 29
    Mandible Dental Regions [1 - 5] ..................................................................... 34
        *Central Region* .......................................................................................... 34
    Canine and Premolar Region (Figs. 50-52) [1 - 5] ............................................ 36
    Molar Region [3 - 5] ....................................................................................... 40
    Periodontium Regions [1 - 5] .......................................................................... 41
    Horizontal and Vertical Bone Loss [1 - 5] ....................................................... 45
    Furcation Involvement [3 - 5] ......................................................................... 49
    Occlusal Radiographs [4 - 5] .......................................................................... 50

Mandibular Occlusal Technique ............................................................... 53
**CONCLUSION** ................................................................................. 54
**CONSENT FOR PUBLICATION** ................................................. 54
**CONFLICT OF INTEREST** .......................................................... 54
**ACKNOWLEDGEMENTS** ............................................................ 54
**REFERENCES** .............................................................................. 54

**CHAPTER 4 ANATOMY OF EXTRAORAL TECHNIQUES** ............................. 56
*Plauto C. A. Watanabe, Emiko S. Arita, Angela J. Camargo* and *Marina G. Baladi*
**CRANIAL [1 - 4]** ........................................................................... 56
Cross Section of Skull [1 - 4] ............................................................ 56
PA projection – Waters [1 - 4] .......................................................... 63
Frontal View of Skull [1 - 4] ............................................................ 64
Panoramic Radiograph [1 - 4] .......................................................... 65
**CONSENT FOR PUBLICATION** ................................................. 76
**CONFLICT OF INTEREST** .......................................................... 76
**ACKNOWLEDGEMENTS** ............................................................ 76
**REFERENCES** .............................................................................. 76

**CHAPTER 5 PATHOLOGIES AND ANATOMICAL ABNORMALITIES** .................. 77
*Plauto C. A. Watanabe, Emiko S. Arita, Angela J. Camargo* and *Marina G. Baladi*
**QUANTITATIVE CHANGES (NUMBER) [1]** ............................. 77
**SIZE ANOMALIES [1]** ................................................................. 79
**MORPHOLOGICAL CHANGES (SHAPE) [1]** ......................... 80
**ANOMALIES OF STRUCTURE [1]** ........................................... 84
**CONCLUSION** ............................................................................. 84
**CONSENT FOR PUBLICATION** ................................................. 85
**CONFLICT OF INTEREST** .......................................................... 85
**ACKNOWLEDGEMENTS** ............................................................ 85
**REFERENCE** ................................................................................ 85

**SUBJECT INDEX** ................................................................................. 86

# FOREWORD

It is an invaluable privilege to be invited to compose the Preface of this e-Book on "Radiological Anatomy, applied in Diagnostic Imaging" of relevant application and indispensable interest for Dentistry / Medicine. The book is available to the community specialized in Dental and Medical Radiology (and related areas) for undergraduate and graduate students, as well as professionals as general or specialized clinicians and for teachers at any stage of their academic career. The indisputable merit of the Brazilian dental literature in filling gaps that provide an adequate source of up-to-date and qualified knowledge should be highlighted by the dedication, competence and herculean commitment of the associate professors Emiko Saito Arita (FOUSP) and Plauto Christopher Aranha Watanabe (FORP-USP). If arduous research activity is also important to enrich teaching and care, no less significant is to consolidate and socialize the respective knowledge through this book. Between these two approaches, the other chapters deal with various aspects of radiographic techniques that are always dependent on full domain of the craniofacial anatomical bases in procedures with specific diagnostic purposes. In addition to its content, it is possible to emphasize the drafting writing promoting easy and pleasant reading, numerous and careful documentation & comprehensive and updated bibliography. Professors Emiko Saito Arita and Plauto Christopher Aranha Watanabe prove, once again, the respective academic merits that further value the acknowledged distinction enjoyed by the University of São Paulo.

**Prof. Luiz Carlos Pardini**
Ribeirão Preto Dental School
São Paulo University
Brazil

# PREFACE

Dental imaging and radiology is a compulsory discipline in any dental curriculum. We intend with this e-book to include the student of this area, professionals of dentistry and medicine, in a way more digestible to such a generation "Y", besides, of course, to make a more visual reading of the content, with a large amount of images for these professionals. Not by chance, it is an academic didactic material of dental imaging and radiology. Radiography is still the main diagnostic tool for dentistry and often for medicine. Thus, all the specialties and the general practitioner make routine use of this examination, aiming to collect, observe and interpret data for the construction of the diagnosis. We will address the subject at the basic / intermediate level, which will certainly include the specialty, professionals and also the graduate. This academic didactic material will be covered in basic (more technical) radiology and also in diagnostic radiology (radiographic interpretation). It is our proposal to primarily target this content to the internationally recommended profile, that is, to contribute to the training of health professionals, with a generalist, humanistic, critical and reflexive education, to act at all levels of health care, based on rigor Technical and scientific, always emphasizing that in teaching, theory is inseparable from practice.

**Plauto Christopher Aranha Watanabe**
School of Dentistry of Ribeirão Preto,
University of São Paulo, São Paulo,
Brazil

# List of Contributors

**Angela J. Camargo**    School of Dentistry of Ribeirão Preto, University of São Paulo, São Paulo, Brazil

**Emiko S. Arita**    School of Dentistry of University of São Paulo, São Paulo, Brazil

**Marina G. Baladi**    School of Dentistry of University of São Paulo, São Paulo, Brazil

**Plauto C. A. Watanabe**    School of Dentistry of Ribeirão Preto, University of São Paulo, São Paulo, Brazil

**CHAPTER 1**

# Basic Aspects of Dental Radiographic Images

**Plauto C. A. Watanabe***, **Emiko S. Arita**, **Angela J. Camargo** and **Marina G. Baladi**

*School of Dentistry of Ribeirão Preto, University of São Paulo, São Paulo, Brazil*

**Abstract:** Anatomical study of skull and face bones is complex and is important in understanding these structures to obtain correct radiographic projections, radiographic findings and interpretation of these images. Modern diagnostic image offers a wide range of methods and techniques, allowing us to study the function and craniofacial morphology in detail, regardless of projection. X-rays emerge as a diverging cone beam from the source and the image produced is composed of multiple superimposed structures.

**Keywords:** Anatomy, Dental radiography, Facial bones, Radiography, Skull.

## INTRODUCTION [1]

Anatomical structures in this e-book are radiographically visible in conventional radiographs, which are clinically important. The book is dedicated to study anatomical structures as a basis for understanding the pathology.

The interpretation of radiographs requires a careful approach. The person responsible for radiographic interpretation should undertake a systematic review of radiographs. This requires detailed analysis of bone structure as well as soft tissue, known areas of complex anatomy and periphery of the film whose condition may be only partially shown, when making necessary complementation.

The decision to conduct a radiographic examination is based on the individual patient characteristics. These include age, general health, clinical findings, dental and systemic history. Radiographic examination is required when the history and clinical examination do not show enough information to fully assess the patient's condition and develop an appropriate treatment plan.

---

* **Corresponding author Plauto C. A. Watanabe:** School of Dentistry of Ribeirão Preto, University of São Paulo, São Paulo, Brazil; Tel: 55-16-33153993; E-mail: watanabe@forp.usp.br

## IDEAL RADIOGRAPH

The ideal radiographic image should have the maximum possible quality, same size and shape of the object, optimal definition / detail, appropriate density and contrast. The anatomical accuracy should have maximum definition and minimal distortion (Fig. **1**).

The terms used to describe the radiographic images are standardized in academic circles. The radiolucency represents the shades of gray to black, the images appear darker in the radiography, therefore it represents low density of the radiographed object (airways, soft tissues, *etc*.) (Fig. **2**).

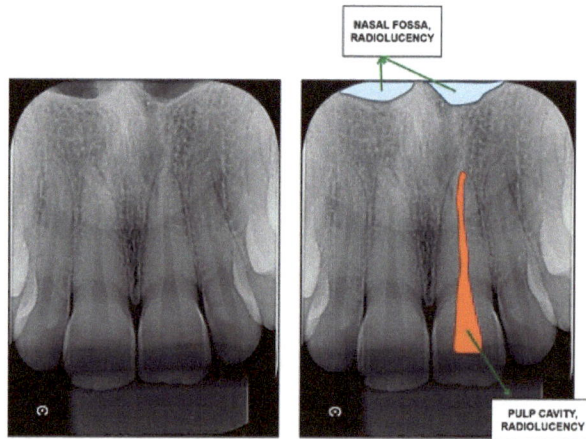

**Fig. (1).** Radiolucency areas.

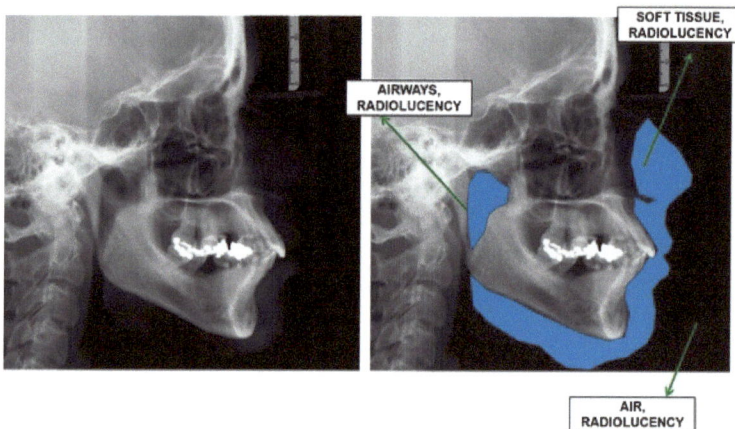

**Fig. (2).** Radiolucency areas.

The radiopacity represents from the color white to the shades of gray, the images appear clearer in the radiography, therefore it represents high density or high atomic number of the radiographed object (metal structures, enamel, osseous cortical, *etc.*) (Fig. **3**)

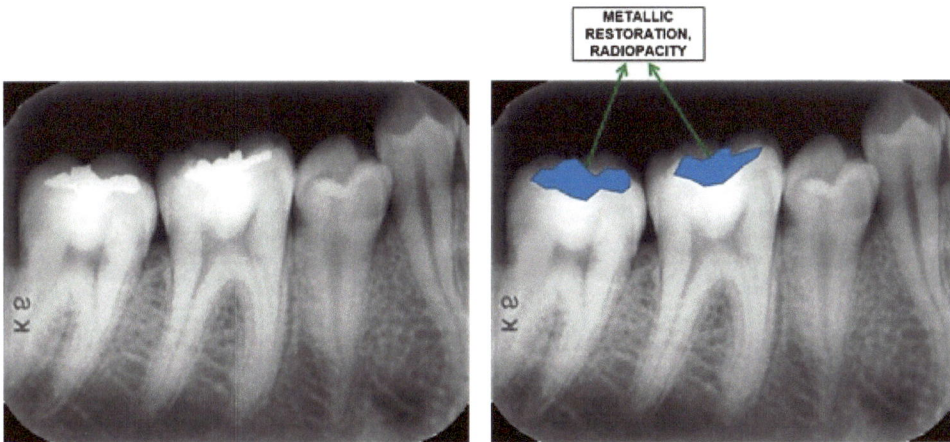

**Fig. (3).** Radiopacity areas.

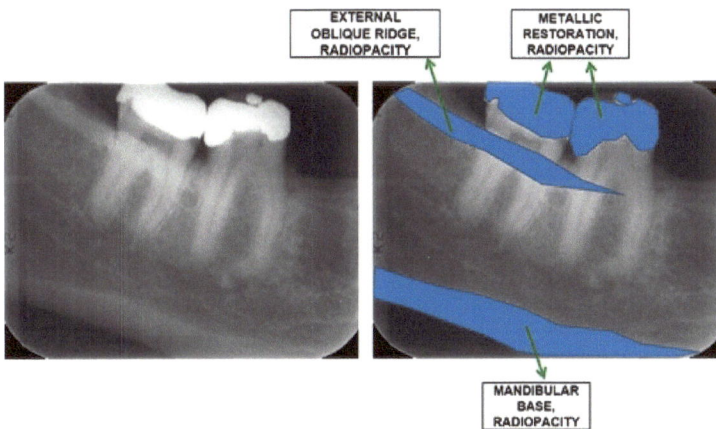

**Fig. (4).** Radiopacity areas.

The radiographic density indicates the degree of darkening. Another widely used term is radiographic contrast, which indicates differences in object densities, and is classified as a short scale when it has less variation of tones and the long scale with a greater variation of tones. The definition of the radiographic image must have the exact delimitation of the anatomical structures of the radiography (Fig. **4**).

All factors: density, contrast, definition and distortion interfere with the radiographic quality and the process of image formation.

## CONCLUSION

For correct interpretation of the radiographic images, shadows recorded in radiographic films and / or electronic records (Plates of phosphorus or CCD / CMOS) it is primordial the knowledge of the anatomical structures of region and the incidence of the central beam of X - rays.

## CONSENT FOR PUBLICATION

Not applicable.

## CONFLICT OF INTEREST

Radiographic material of the NACEDO - Nucleus of Support to Culture and Extension in Dental Diagnosis of the Pro-Rectory of Culture and University Extension (PRCExU / USP). Crowded at the School of Dentistry of Ribeirão Preto / University of São Paulo.

## ACKNOWLEDGEMENTS

NACEDO-PRCExU/USP

## REFERENCE

[1]     Watanabe PC, Arita ES. Radiologia Odontológica e Imaginologia. 1st ed., Rio de Janeiro: Elsevier 2012.

# CHAPTER 2

# Dental Radiographic Techniques

**Plauto C. A. Watanabe***, **Emiko S. Arita**, **Angela J. Camargo** and **Marina G. Baladi**

*School of Dentistry of Ribeirão Preto, University of São Paulo, São Paulo, Brazil*

**Abstract:** Dental radiographic techniques include intra- and extraoral techniques. Among the intraoral techniques, the most used are the bisector technique and the interproximal technique. These are the radiographic techniques that produce greater sharpness or details of the image of the dental structures, with the exception of CTBC. The extraoral radiographic technique most commonly used in the dental routine is the panoramic radiograph, since it encompasses the entire maxillo-mandibular complex, the teeth naturally, and neighboring structures.

**Keywords:** Extraoral radiography, Intraoral radiography, Interproximal, Panoramic, Periapical.

## INTRAORAL EXAMINATIONS [1 - 3]

Intraoral radiography is performed with the introduction of a dental film or a digital device into the oral cavity in the region of the tooth to be evaluated. This technique produces a highly sharp radiographic image (teeth and supporting structures), is a low-cost examination and has low radiation dose.

### Periapical Radiography

Periapical radiography (PpR) has the main objective of visualizing the tooth or group of teeth in their integrality and their support structures. A free margin of the occlusal / incisal surfaces should be left to avoid crown cuts (3-5 mm) and also beyond the apex of the teeth (5 mm) to analyze the health of the bone tissue (Fig. **1**).

In periapical radiographs, the angle between the long axis of the tooth and the long axis of the radiographic film / sensor due to dental-maxillo-mandibular anatomy should be taken into account. (Fig. **2**).

* **Corresponding author Plauto C. A. Watanabe:** School of Dentistry of Ribeirão Preto, University of São Paulo, São Paulo, Brazil; Tel: 55-16-33153993; E-mail: watanabe@forp.usp.br

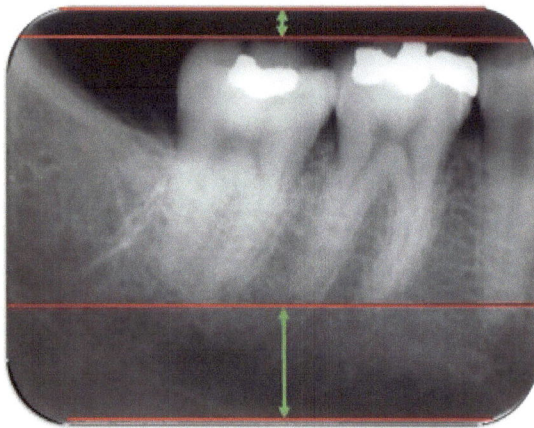

**Fig. (1).** A free margin of the occlusal / incisal surfaces should be left to avoid crown cuts (3-5 mm) and also beyond the apex of the teeth (5 mm) to analyze the health of the bone tissue.

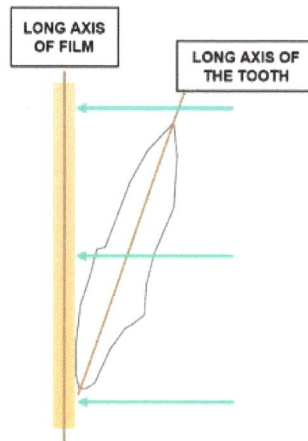

**Fig. (2).** Radiographic film / sensor and tooth relation: real condition without use of positioners, causing object distortion.

The periapical radiographs are performed in all groups of teeth, and the whole mouth exam (14 radiographs) is widely used for periodontal evaluation (Fig. **3**). To realize this technique, it is necessary to use the positioners (RINN® and HANSHIN® type) that act through the parallelism reducing the distortion of the object.

## Interproximal Radiography (Bite-wing)

The interproximal technique (Fig. **4**) is widely used for the assessment of interdental contact points. Interproximal radiographs record the images of the limits, positions and contours of the crowns (upper and lower teeth), as well as the alveolar bone crest and the coronary portion of the roots. The presence of caries in these regions is more evident in this technique. In these dental regions, other techniques available may generate overlapping structures.

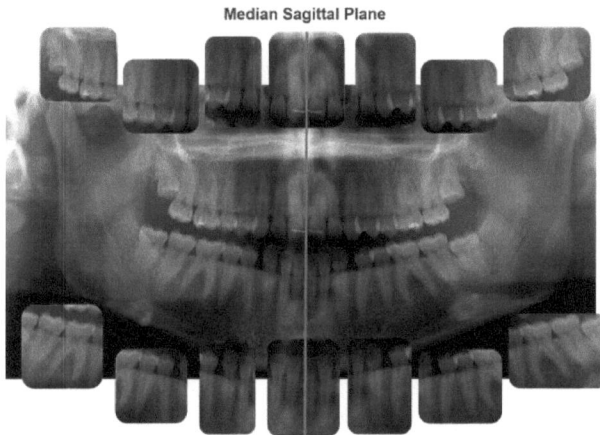

**Fig. (3).** Division of radiographic films by dental regions for the whole mouth exam.

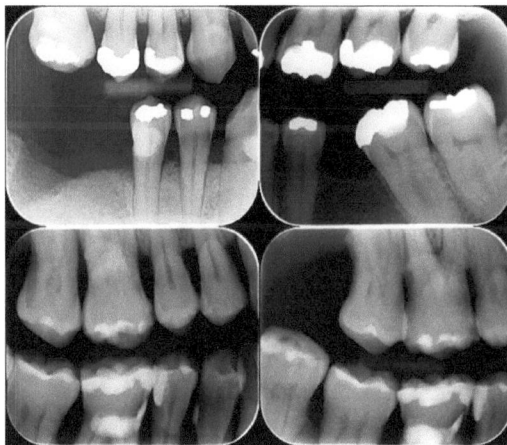

**Fig. (4).** Division of radiographic films by dental regions for interproximal/bite-wing exam.

## Occlusal Radiography

Occlusal radiography is obtained by positioning the radiographic film/sensor parallel to the occlusal surfaces of teeth or alveolar ridge. It can be performed on the maxilla and mandible (Fig. **5**). The film used for this technique is larger than the previous techniques. It is used for alveolar ridge analysis for prosthetic evaluation, research of included teeth, anatomical abnormalities, foreign bodies, *etc*.

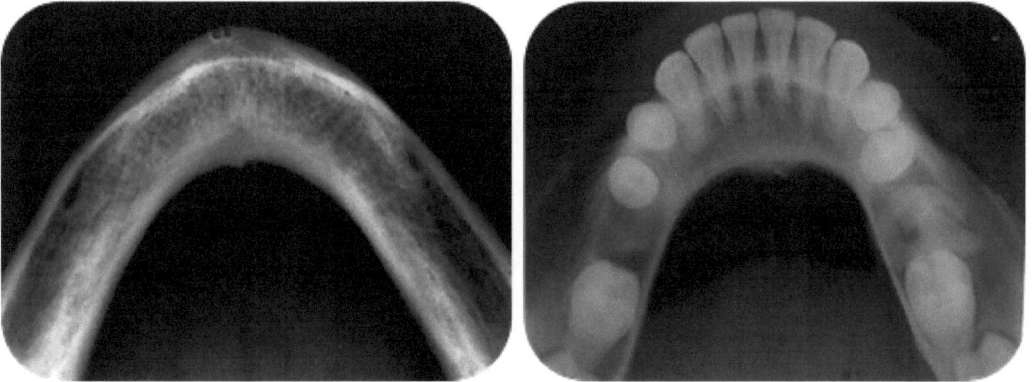

**Fig. (5).** Occlusal radiography performed on the mandible.

## EXTRAORAL EXAMINATIONS [1 - 3]

In routine dental care, intraoral radiographic examinations are most commonly used due to practicality (minor equipment) and small areas of analysis. However, when there is a need to analyze the surrounding structures of the oral cavity, there are other tests called extraoral.

### Panoramic Radiography

Panoramic radiography (PR) occupies second place in importance behind intraoral radiography. PR imaging (Fig. **6**) may be of more benefit to patients by providing excellent visibility of anatomical structures, assessment of the maxillary sinus region, evaluation of mandible fractures, and tooth development. It also has the additional benefit of radiation dose reduction as compared to whole mouth intraoral radiographs.

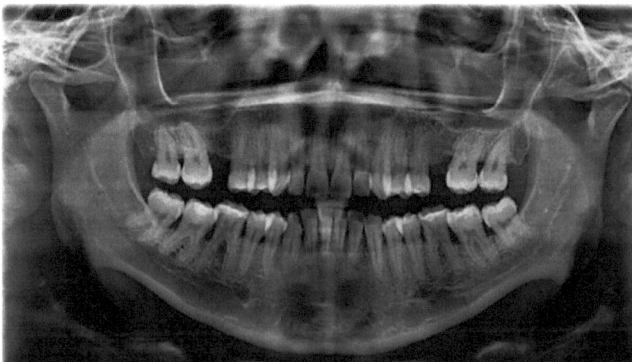

**Fig. (6).** Panoramic Radiography.

The PR is versatile because it can evaluate different areas of the head. Depending on the cut used, it is possible to evaluate the maxillary sinuses and temporomandibular joint (TMJ).

## Temporomandibular Joint Radiography (Transcranial)

TMJ radiography (Fig. **7**) use for the analysis of temporomandibular dysfunction is limited, but it is requested in the clinical routine for ease access to this examination. It is used for evaluation of fracture with displacement of the fragments, morphological alterations, evaluation of bone structures (head of mandible, mandibular fossa and articular eminence), trauma and pathological processes. The most suitable for evaluation of TMJ (bone and soft tissue) is the magnetic resonance imaging (MRI).

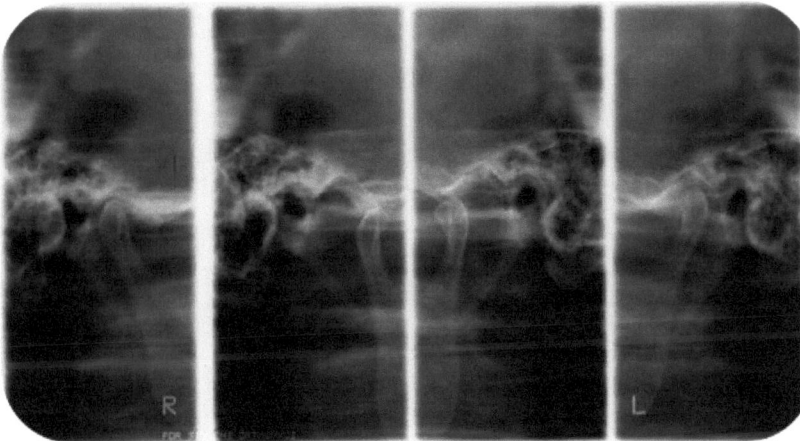

**Fig. (7).** Temporomandibular Joint Radiography.

## Cephalometric Radiography

These are exams that cover the head and neck region, can be performed mostly in panoramic radiography equipment with cephalometric arm.

## Teleradiograph (Lateral)

Teleradiograph is widely used in orthodontics and orthognathic surgeries, because with the aid of cephalostat device, radiographic shots can be standardized (Fig. **8**). Proper patient positioning is essential for the study of craniofacial development. Radiographic cephalometry is performed from this examination with the measurement of human head dimensions.

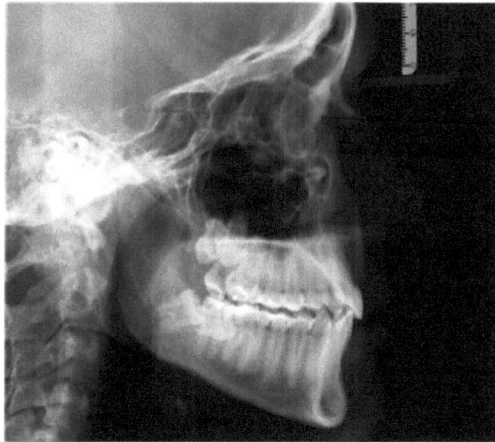

**Fig. (8).** Teleradiograph with cephalostat device.

## PA Skull

It is the projection technique in the occipital-frontal direction (Fig. **9**). There are several modifications of this technique. It is indicated to evaluate the facial growth (Ricketts analysis), trauma, pathologies, analysis of the sinuses, orbits, nasal cavity and facial symmetry.

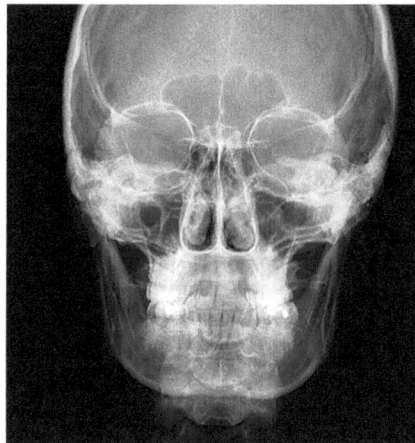

**Fig. (9).** PA Skull.

## PA Projection (Waters)

Projection technique in the PA direction, also called Waters projection (Fig. **10**). Used for evaluation of the maxillary sinuses (comparative between the sides), frontal and ethmoid, the orbits, frontozygomatic suture and nasal cavity.

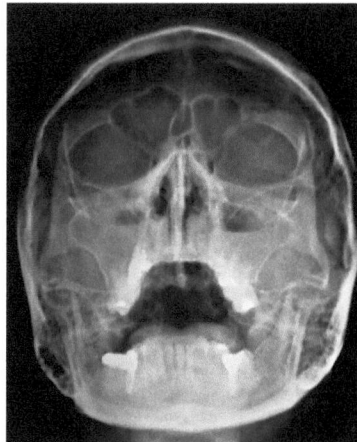

**Fig. (10).** PA projection (Waters).

## Axial (Hirtz Projection)

It is a technique that aims to evaluate the base of the skull, jaw heads, coronoid process, sphenoid sinus, mandible curvature, lateral / posterior wall of the maxillary sinuses and displacement of possible fracture of the zygomatic arch (Fig. **11**).

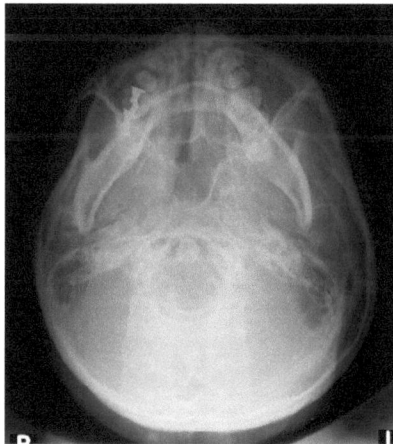

**Fig. (11).** Axial (Hirtz Projection).

## CONCLUSION

Different radiographic techniques or X - ray incidence on the different structures for analysis can provide three - dimensional (3D) images, when associate 2 or more of these techniques, considering different points of entry for X - rays and different beam angulations.

## CONSENT FOR PUBLICATION

Not applicable.

## CONFLICT OF INTEREST

Radiographic material of the NACEDO - Nucleus of Support to Culture and Extension in Dental Diagnosis of the Pro-Rectory of Culture and University Extension (PRCExU / USP). Crowded at the School of Dentistry of Ribeirão Preto / University of São Paulo.

## ACKNOWLEDGEMENTS

NACEDO-PRCExU/USP

## REFERENCES

[1]     Langland OE, Langlais RP. Princípios do diagnostico por imagem em Odontologia. 1st ed., Português 2002.

[2]     Watanabe PC, Arita ES. Radiologia Odontológica e Imaginologia. 1st ed., Rio de Janeiro: Elsevier 2012.

[3]     Yiu B-K, Chi-Man S, Chi-Yung Liu S, Chi-Hong P, Hin-Ho Siu G. Digital dental panoramic radiography: evaluation of image quality in four imaging systems. Hong Kong Dental Journal 2005; 2: 19-23.

# CHAPTER 3

# Anatomy of Intraoral Techniques

**Plauto C. A. Watanabe\***, **Emiko S. Arita**, **Angela J. Camargo** and **Marina G. Baladi**

*School of Dentistry of Ribeirão Preto, University of São Paulo, São Paulo, Brazil*

**Abstract:** Anatomy (from the ancient Greek anatomy, "section"), is the branch of biology in which the structure and organization of living beings are studied, both externally and internally (http://en.wikipedia.org/wiki/Anatomia). All species / structures have characteristics that are inherent, which are normal to them. For the recognition of these normal structures of the teeth and other structures of the maxillo-mandibular complex, seen as projection of radiographic shadows, it is necessary to have prior knowledge of equivalent morphophysiology, besides the knowledge of dental radiographic techniques. In order to be able to indicate the pathological state, and / or abnormal, one must know the radiographic image of the normal anatomical structure correctly. It is important to recognize the normal anatomical structure, among the radiolucent and radiopaque images of the maxillo-mandibular complex.

**Keywords:** Dental anatomy, Maxillo-mandibular complex.

## PERIAPICAL AND INTERPROXIMAL RADIOGRAPHS [1 - 5]

### Dental Regions

ENAMEL was radiographically identified as well-defined radiopaque image, covering the entire crown, with thickness tapering to the extent that approaches the cervical margin, where it ends. The degree of enamel radiopacity, respecting the variations in thickness, is one of the most important signals to the clinical research as dental caries, especially the interproximal (Fig. **1**).

DENTIN is radiographically presented as less radiopaque than the enamel. It represents the larger portion of the hard tooth tissues and less calcified (Figs. **2** and **3**).

\* **Corresponding author Plauto C. A. Watanabe:** School of Dentistry of Ribeirão Preto, University of São Paulo, São Paulo, Brazil; Tel: 55-16-33153993; E-mail: watanabe@forp.usp.br

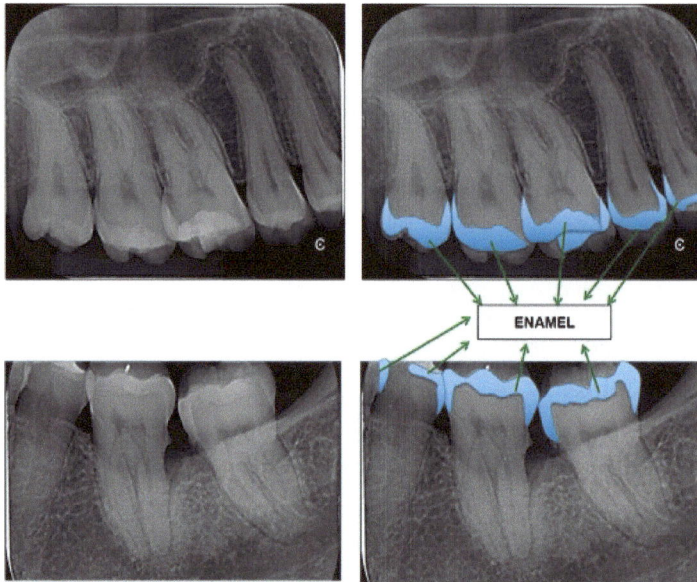

**Fig. (1).** Superior and inferior molar periapical radiography with featured Enamel.

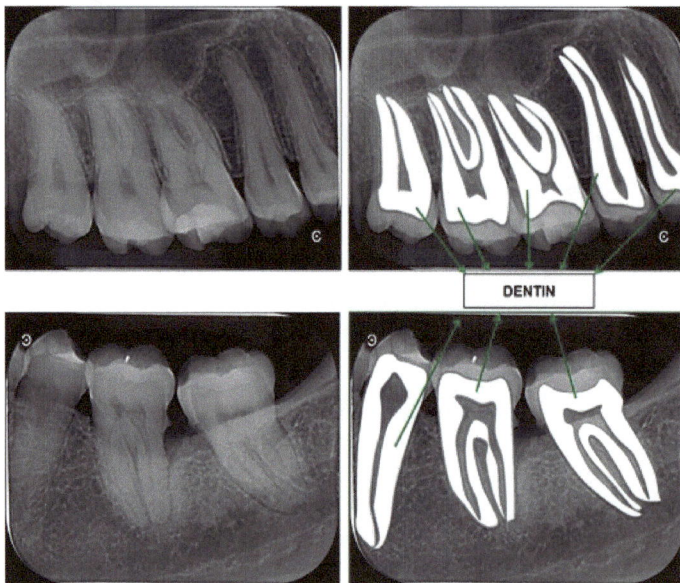

**Fig. (2).** Superior and inferior molar periapical radiography with featured Dentin.

PULP CAVITY - it is seen radiographically as a radiolucent image occupying the center of tooth (coronal portion) and extending to the tooth apex (root canal), due to its high permeability to X-rays. The topography varies according to tooth (Figs. **4** and **5**).

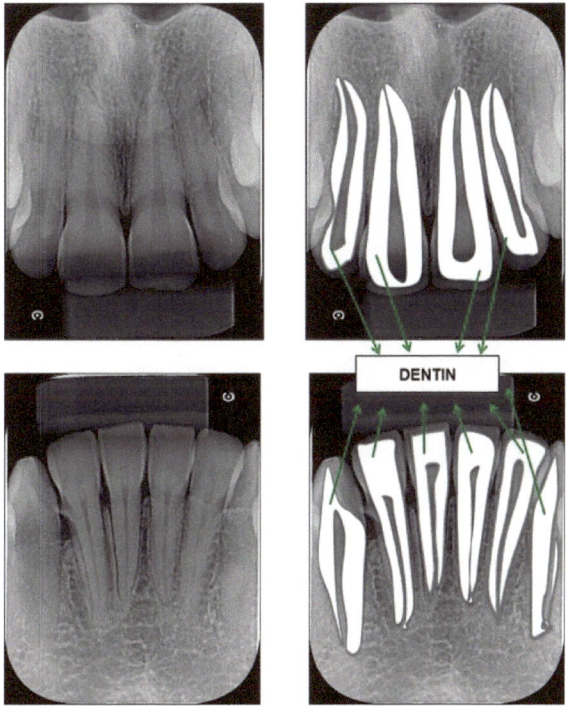

**Fig. (3).** Superior and inferior incisor periapical radiography with featured Dentin.

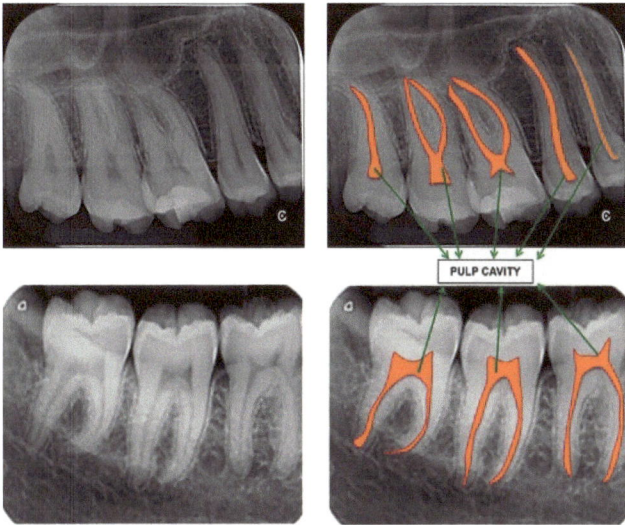

**Fig. (4).** Superior and inferior molar periapical radiography with featured Pulp Cavity.

CEMENT appears under normal conditions as a thin structure, making it impossible for it to be radiographically distinguishable from dentin saved in cases hyperplasia (Figs. **6-11**).

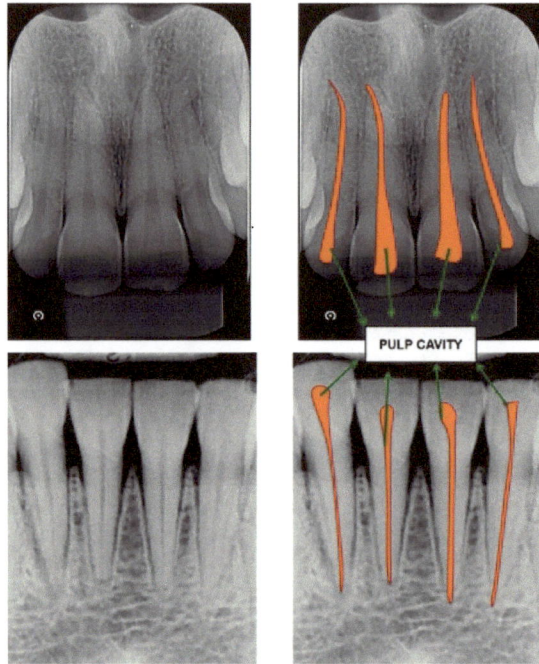

**Fig. (5).** Superior and inferior incisor periapical radiography with featured Pulp Cavity.

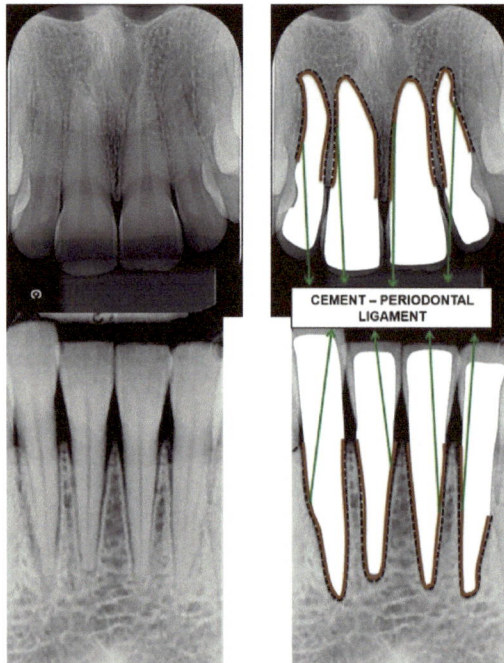

**Fig. (6).** Superior and inferior incisor periapical radiography with featured Cement and periodontal ligament.

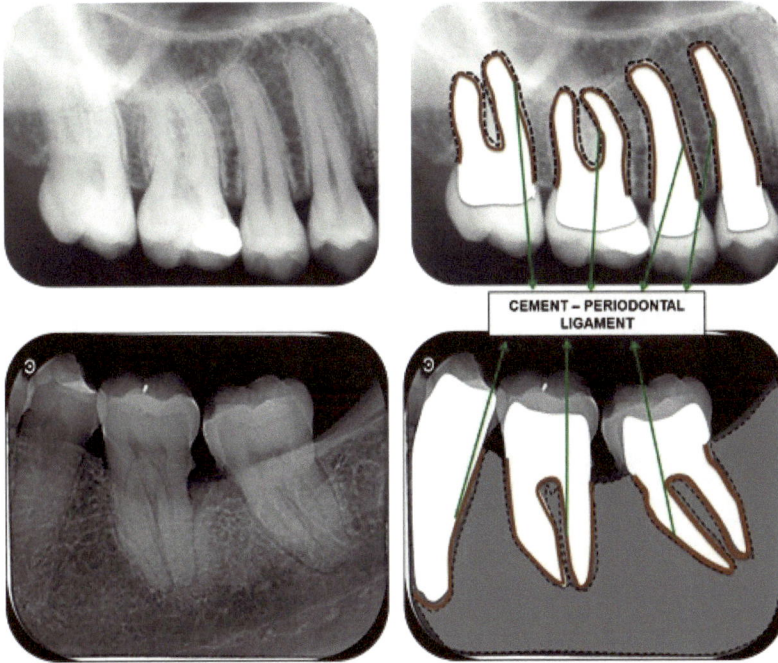

**Fig. (7).** Superior and inferior molar periapical radiography with featured Cement and periodontal ligament.

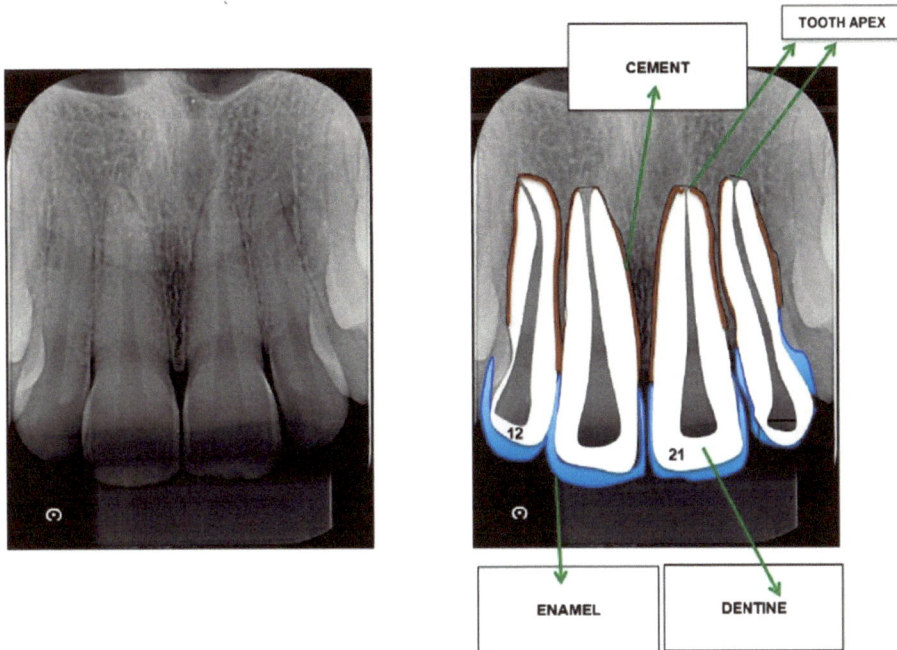

**Fig. (8).** Superior incisor periapical radiography.

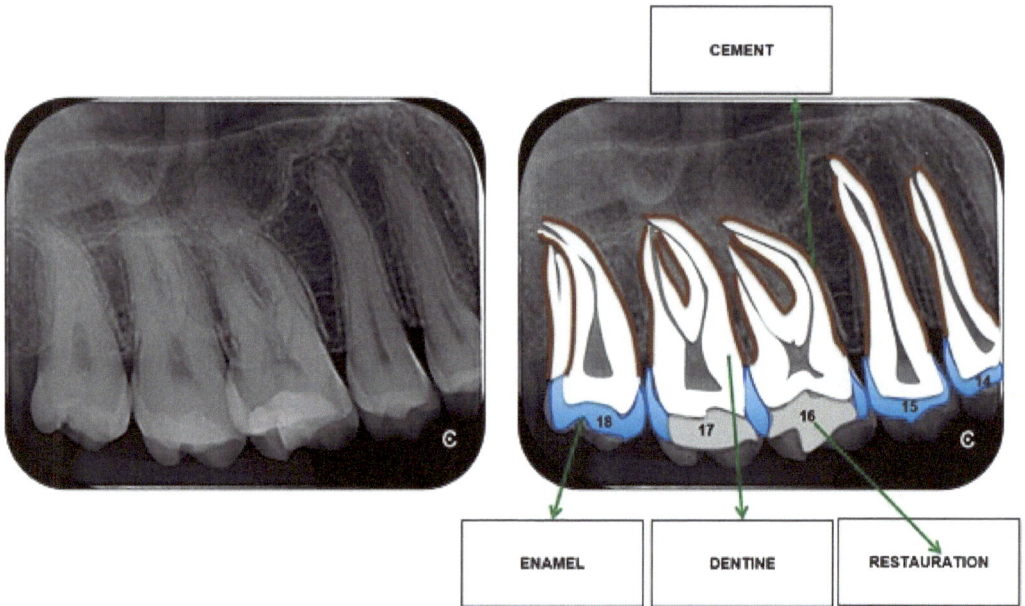

**Fig. (9).** Superior molar periapical radiography.

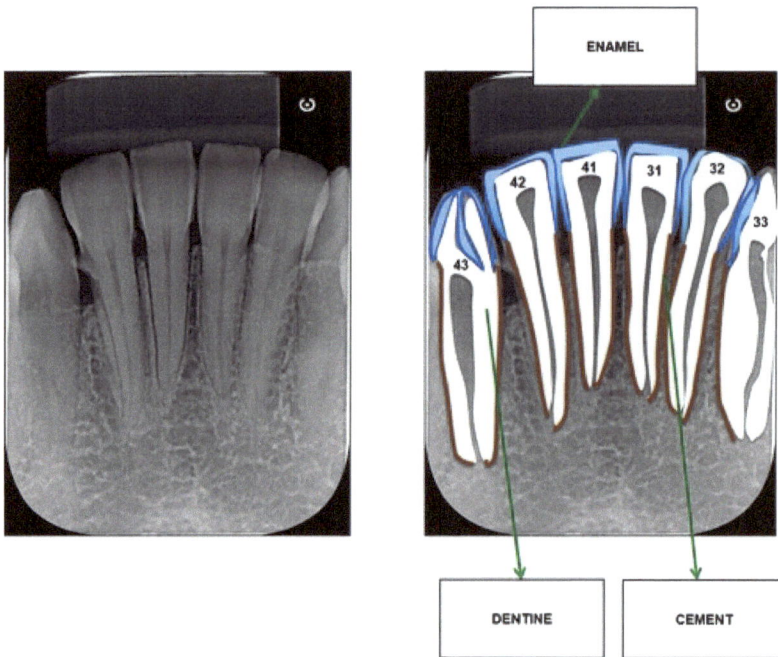

**Fig. (10).** Inferior incisor periapical radiography.

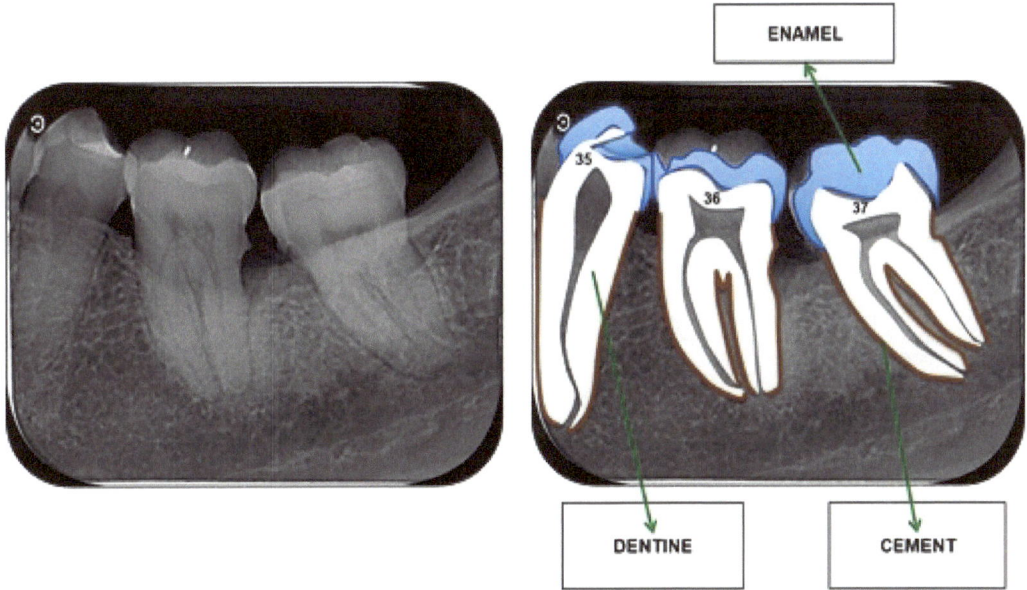

**Fig. (11).** Inferior molar periapical radiography.

LAMINA DURA - radiographically radiopaque appears as a continuous line, the cortical bone surrounding the root portion of the teeth (Figs. **12-14**, **50** and **51**).

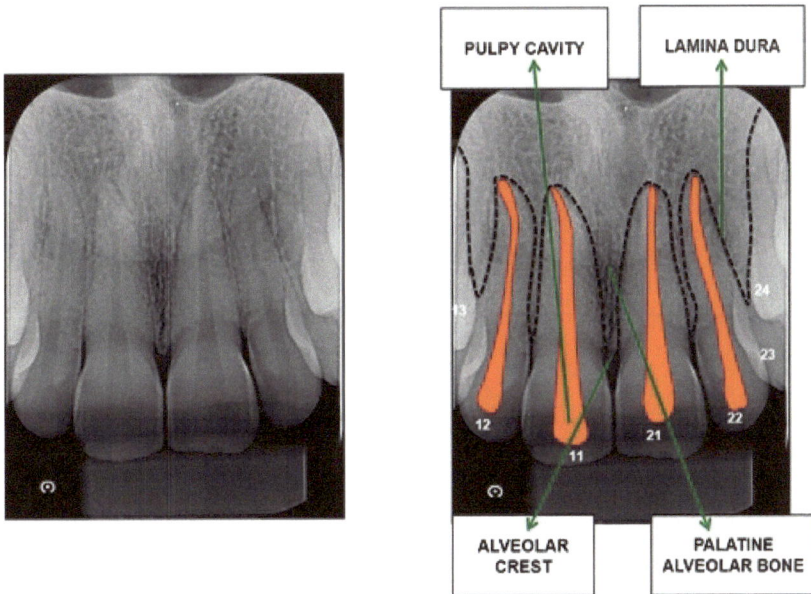

**Fig. (12).** Superior incisor periapical radiography.

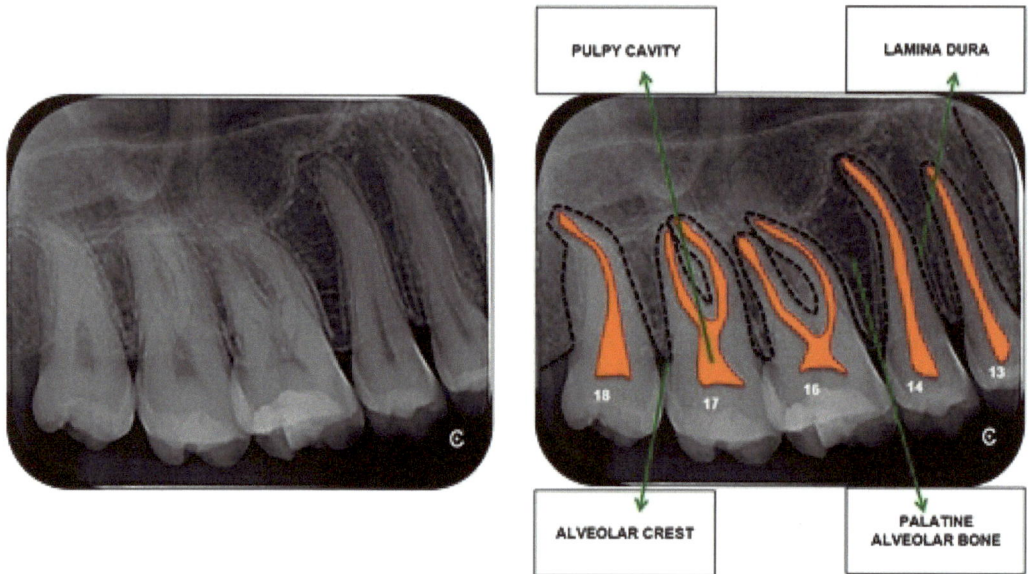

**Fig. (13).** Superior molar periapical radiography.

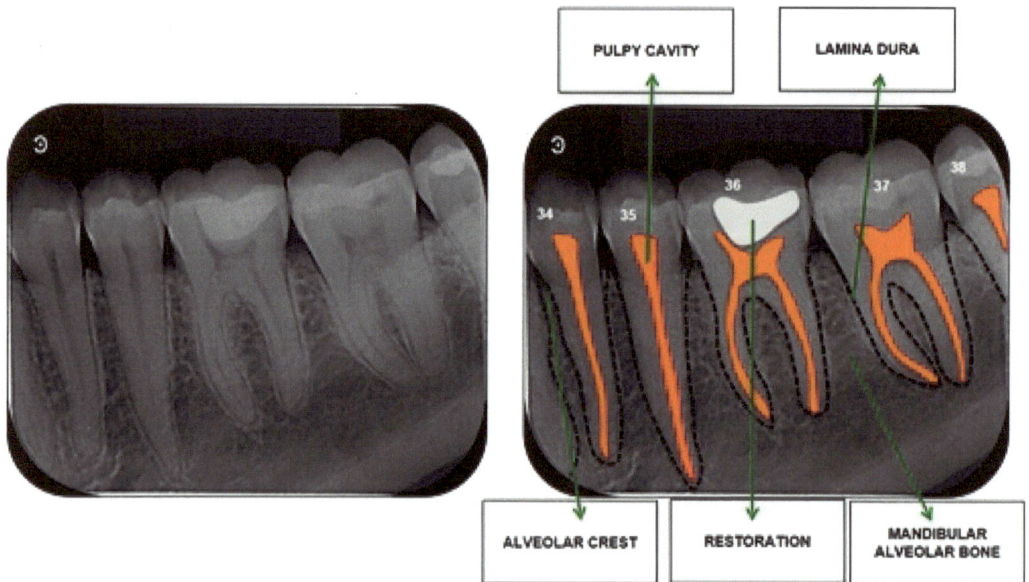

**Fig. (14).** Inferior molar periapical radiography.

PERIODONTAL SPACE - is identified radiographically as a thin radiolucent line skirting the dental root in all the borders or periphery, is the space occupied by the periodontal tissue (Figs. **6**, **7**).

ALVEOLAR BONE CREST - radiographically appears as a radiopaque structure, between a tooth and the other and have bevel shape, gently sloping or straight. It is the continuity of lamina dura forming the alveolar bone crest (Figs. **12-14**, **50**, **51**).

ALVEOLAR BONE - radiographically appears as radiopaque trabeculae bone, limited by radiolucent marrow spaces (Figs. **12-14**).

## Central Region of Maxilla [1 - 5]

INCISIVE FORAMEN appears radiographically between the central incisors or slightly above those in the midline as an oval radiolucent image. Externally, it has the incisive canal bordered by two other radiolucent lines with variables width and length, externally bounded by two other radiopaque lines, which are the record of their sidewalls, terminating at the anterior palatine foramen (incisive foramen). In some cases, a radiographic image overlaps with the apex of central or lateral incisor and can be mistaken for a periapical lesion (Fig. **15**).

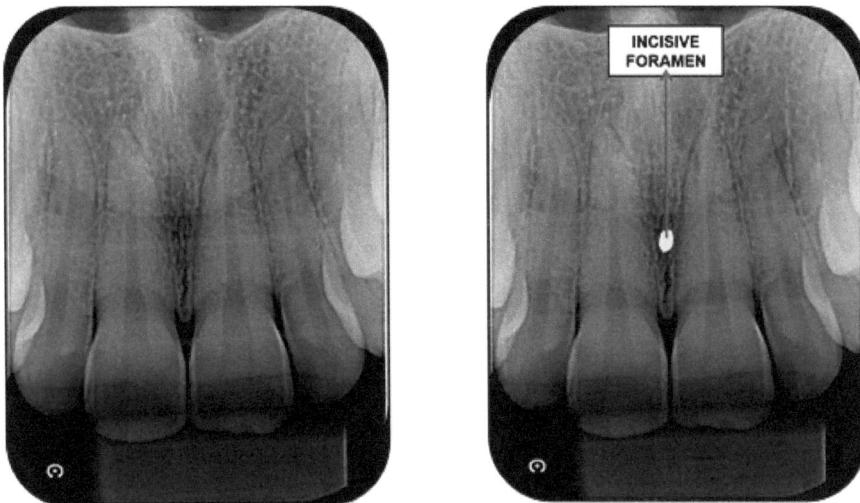

**Fig. (15).** Superior incisor periapical radiography with featured Incisive Foramen.

NASAL CAVITY - in the periapical radiographs of superior central region, they appear as two radiolucent images, symmetrically arranged above the upper incisors and are separated by a thick radiopaque line, which extends to the floor of them, corresponding to the nasal septum (VOMER) (Fig. **16**).

FLOOR OF NASAL FOSSA - can extend to the region of the lateral incisor, canine and posterior regions when it overlaps the maxillary sinus (Fig. **17**).

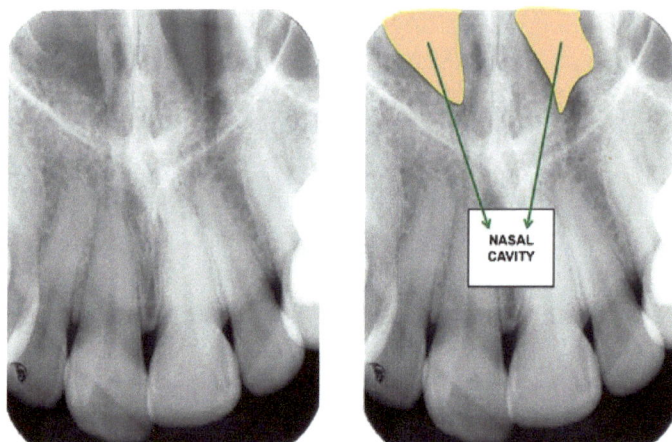

**Fig. (16).** Superior incisor periapical radiography with featured Nasal Cavity.

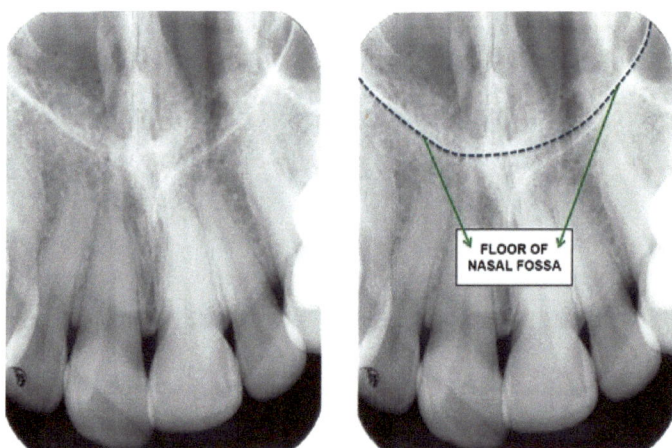

**Fig. (17).** Superior incisor periapical radiography with featured Floor of Nasal Fossa.

SHADOWS OF NOSTRILS - in the periapical radiographs can be observed the overlapping shadow of the nostrils over the alveolar bone, increasing the degree of radiopacity (Fig. **20**).

ANTERIOR NASAL SPINE - in periapical radiographs is observed as a small radiopaque region in a "V" form, corresponding to overlapping of the maxilla at the lower edge of the nasal fossa (Figs. **18-20**).

INTERMAXILLARY SUTURE - observed radiographically as a radiolucent line geometric regularity, is identified especially in young adults, it is not always well defined and could be mistaken for a fracture line, especially in individuals with multiple trauma (Figs. **18-21**).

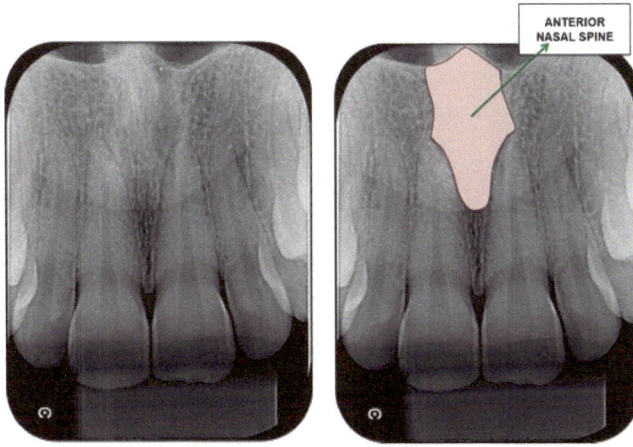

**Fig. (18).** Superior incisor periapical radiography with featured Anterior nasal spine.

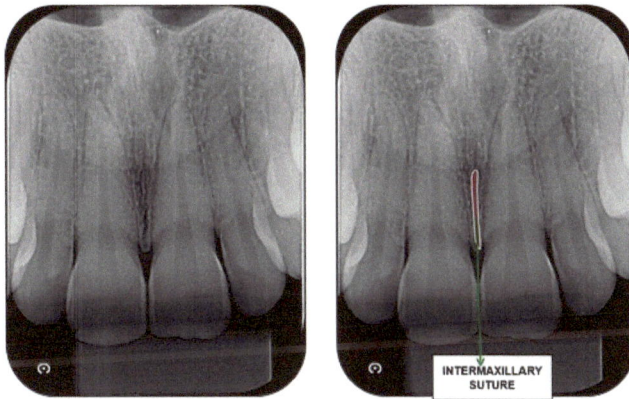

**Fig. (19).** Superior incisor periapical radiography with featured Intermaxillary suture.

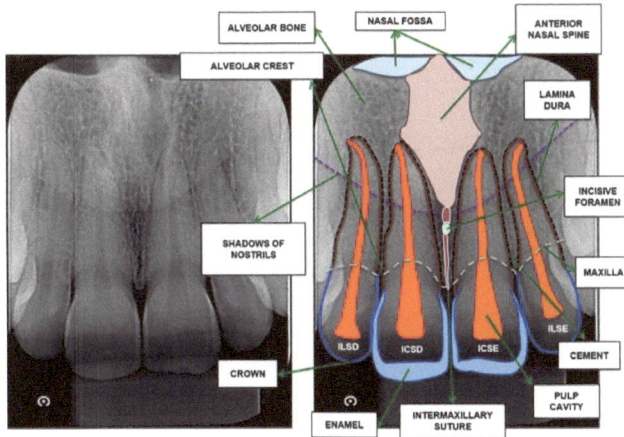

**Fig. (20).** Periapical Radiographs - Superior Incisor Region.

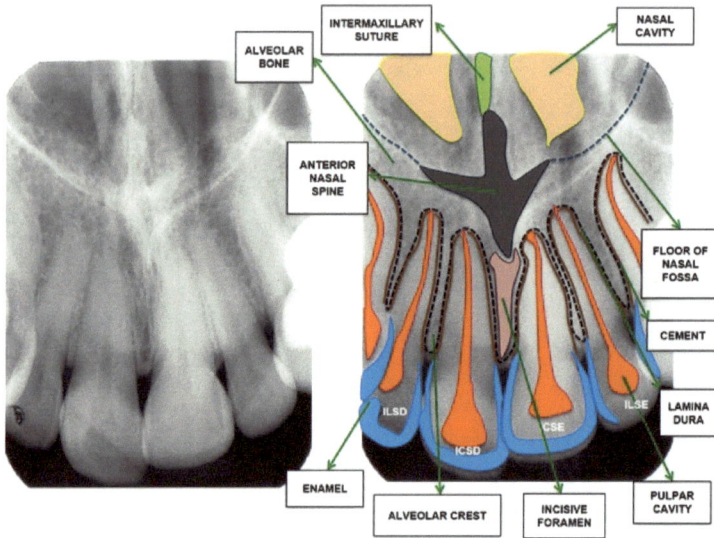

**Fig. (21).** Periapical Radiographs - Superior Incisor Region.

## Lateral Incisor and Canine Region (Fig. 21) [3 - 5]

INCISIVE FOSSAE - radiographically can be seen as an elongated radiolucent region, with variable length and shape, which can be mixed with globule-maxillary cysts. It is located between the canine and the lateral incisor, corresponding to the fovea or a supra-incisal bone depression (Figs. **22-26**).

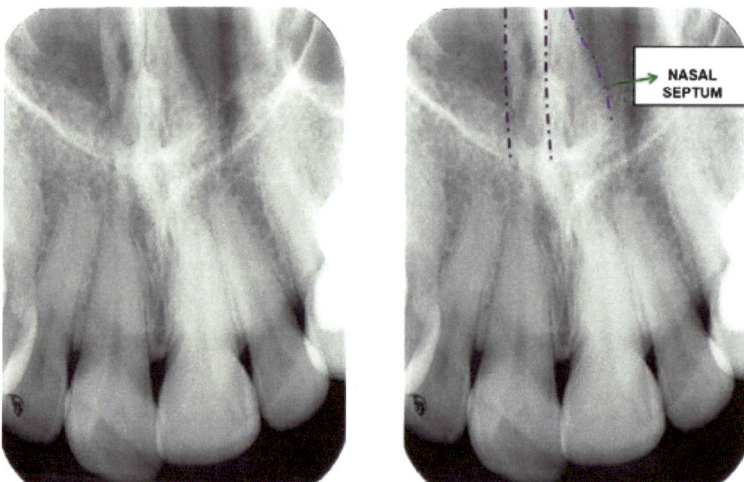

**Fig. (22).** Periapical Radiographs - Lateral Incisor and Canine Region with featured Nasal septum.

SEPTAL - radiographically appear as two radiopaque lines with variable direction and height. Are frequently found looking divide the maxillary sinus in cavities called diverticula (Figs. **22-27**).

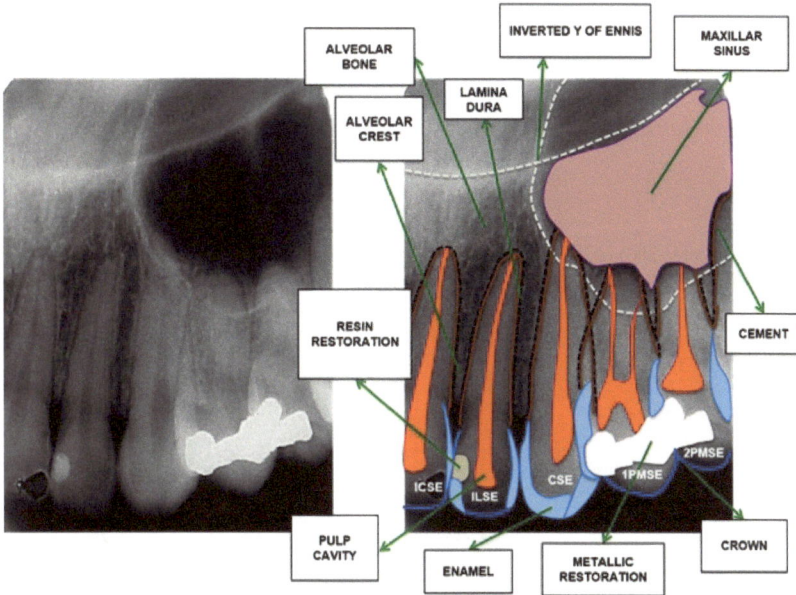

**Fig. (23).** Periapical Radiographs - Lateral Incisor and Canine Region.

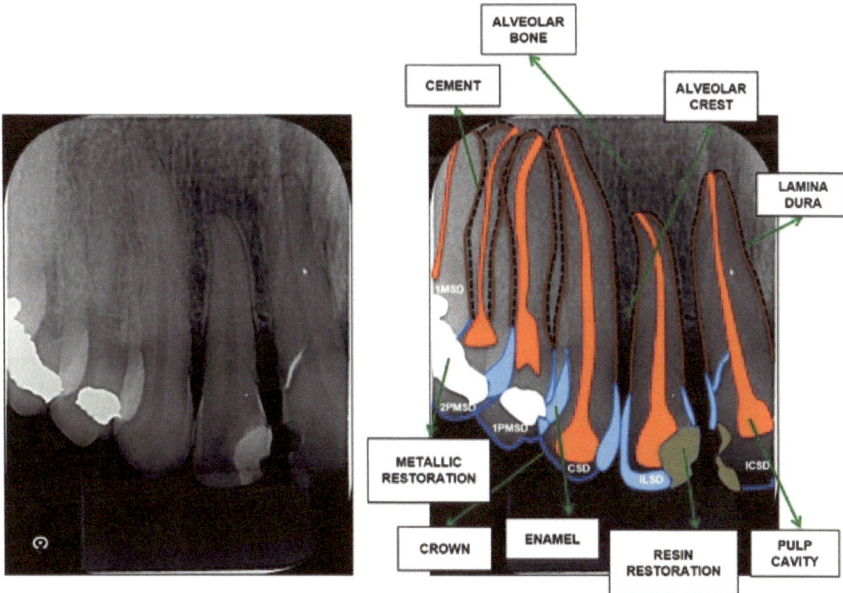

**Fig. (24).** Periapical Radiographs - Lateral Incisor and Canine Region.

NASAL SEPTAL - can be observed radiographically as a radiopaque line in interior of the maxillary sinus. The presence and number of septa inside the maxillary sinus may vary depending on the anatomy of each individual. As shown in (Figs. **23-26**).

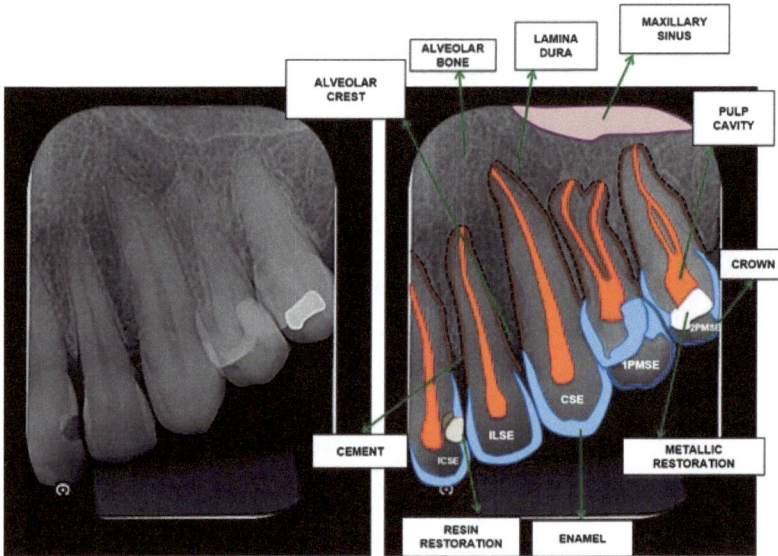

**Fig. (25).** Periapical Radiographs - Lateral Incisor and Canine Region.

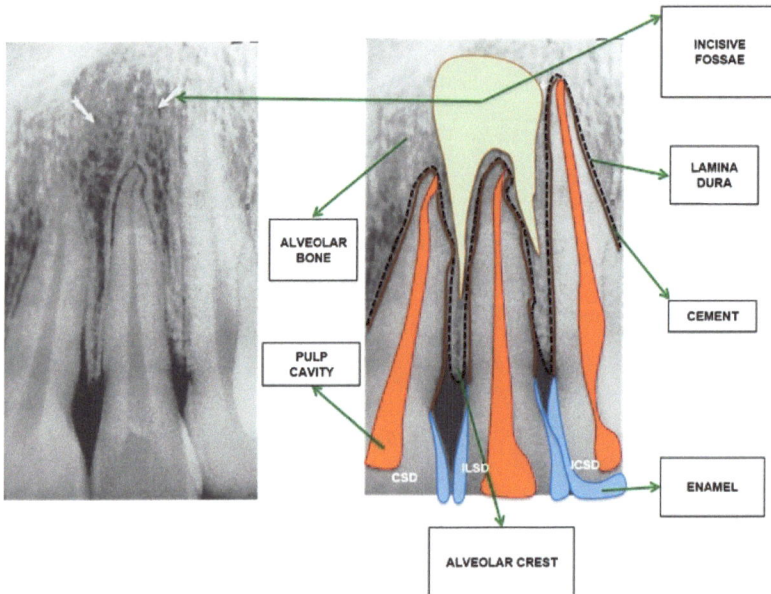

**Fig. (26).** Periapical Radiographs - Lateral Incisor and Canine Region.

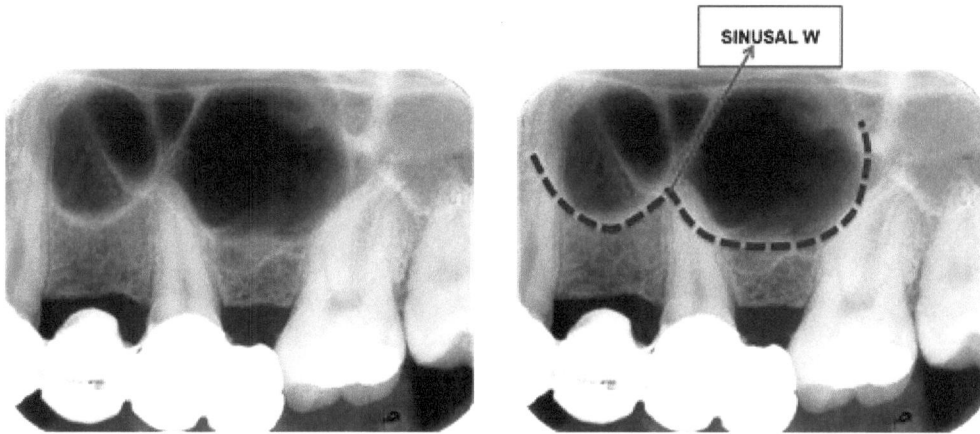

**Fig. (27).** Periapical Radiographs - Canine and Premolar Region with featured Sinusal W.

## Premolar and Molar Region [2 - 5]

SINUS MAXILLARY - it appears radiographically as a radiolucent area located above the Pres molar and molar. The maxillary sinus floor consists of a dense cortical bone and appears as a radiopaque line. The projections can be viewed or its extension, being classified as: 1) Alveolar - develops towards the alveolar bone, frequently observed in cases of absence of molars, reaching the edge. 2) Anterior - develops towards the canine or lateral incisor, the intersection of radiopaque lines corresponding to the floor of the nasal cavity with the anterior wall of the maxillary sinus ("Y" Inverted of Ennis). 3) Toward Maxillary Tuberosity - it is the most common, may take all of the tuberosity, increasing the fragility and enabling fractures in surgery to extraction of third molar teeth. These maxillary sinus extensions are observed radiographically. 4) Palatine - radiographically are more observed in occlusal radiographs, which is characterized by sinus image excavating the floor of the nasal fossa. In edentulous individuals, it is not uncommon to find the zygomatic extension (Figs. **28-31**).

CORTICAL SINUS FORMING THE "W" - radiographically are observed as radiopaque lines inside the maxillary sinus, and aspect "W". The term "sinus W" is used when inside the sinus presenting the presence of a septum.

"Y" INVERTED OF ENNIS - radiographically is viewed as radiopaque lines formed by the intersection of the lateral nasal wall and the anterior edge of the maxillary sinus. Both are composed of dense cortical bone which appears as a radiopaque line. Located above the upper canine.

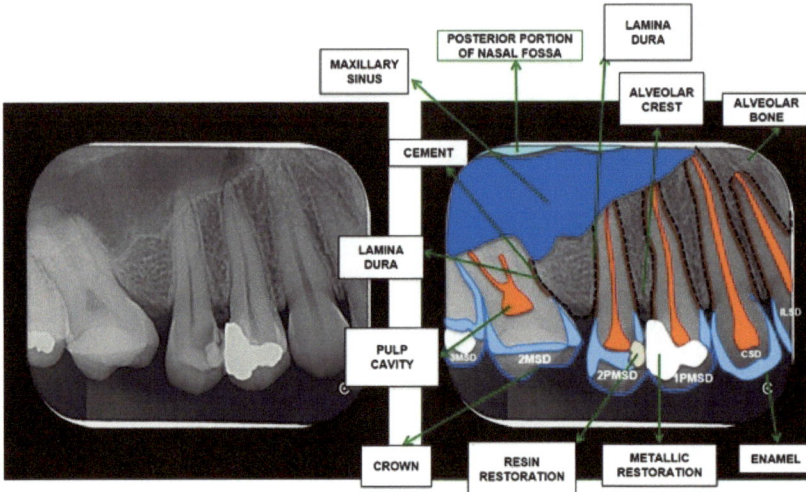

**Fig. (28).** Periapical Radiographs - Canine and Premolar Region.

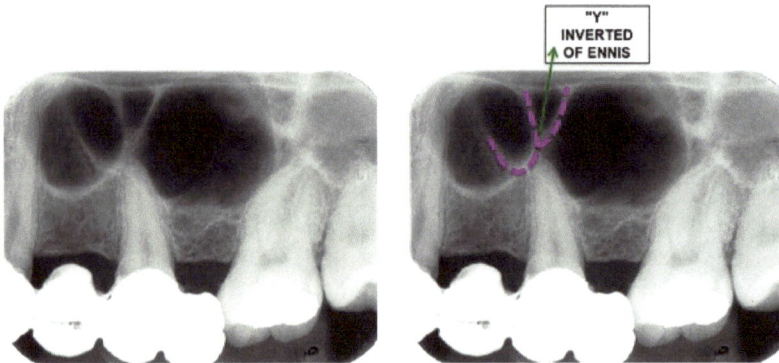

**Fig. (29).** Periapical Radiographs - Premolar and Molar Region with featured "Y" inverted of Ennis..

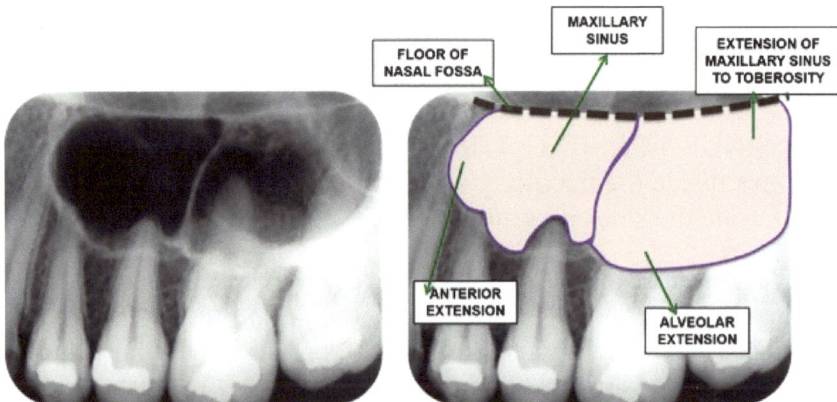

**Fig. (30).** Periapical Radiographs - Premolar and Molar Region.

## Premolar and Molar Region

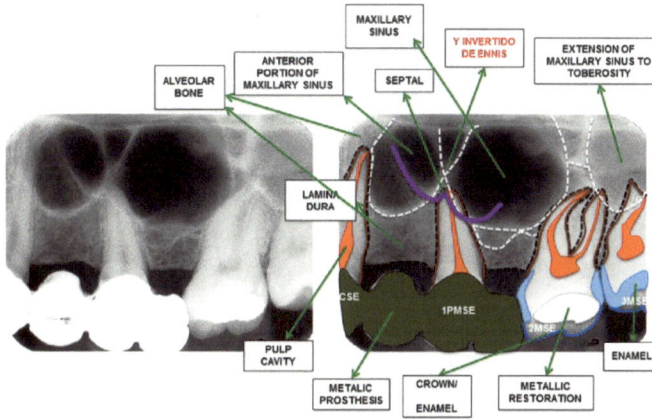

**Fig. (31).** Periapical Radiographs - Premolar and Molar Region.

# Molar Region [1 - 5] (Figs. 32-35)

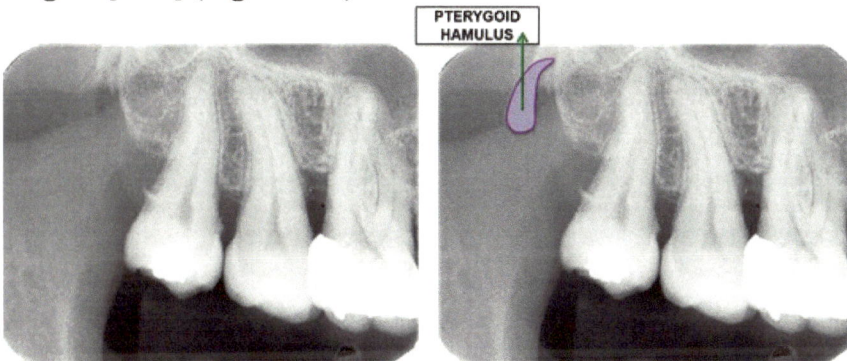

**Fig. (32).** Periapical radiographs - molar region toothless.

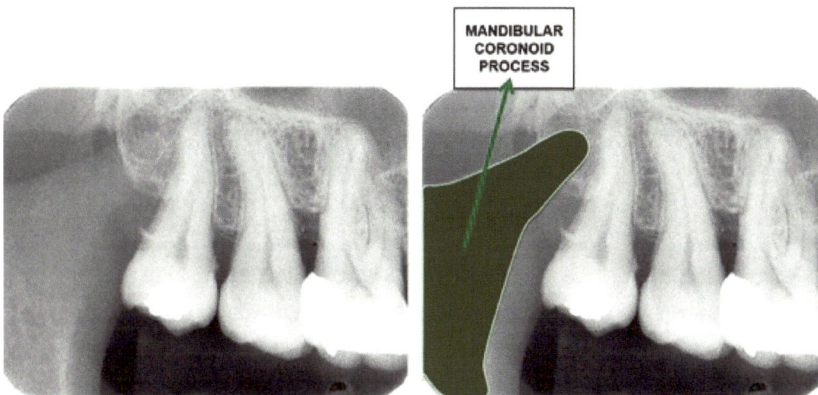

**Fig. (33).** Periapical Radiographs - Molar Region.

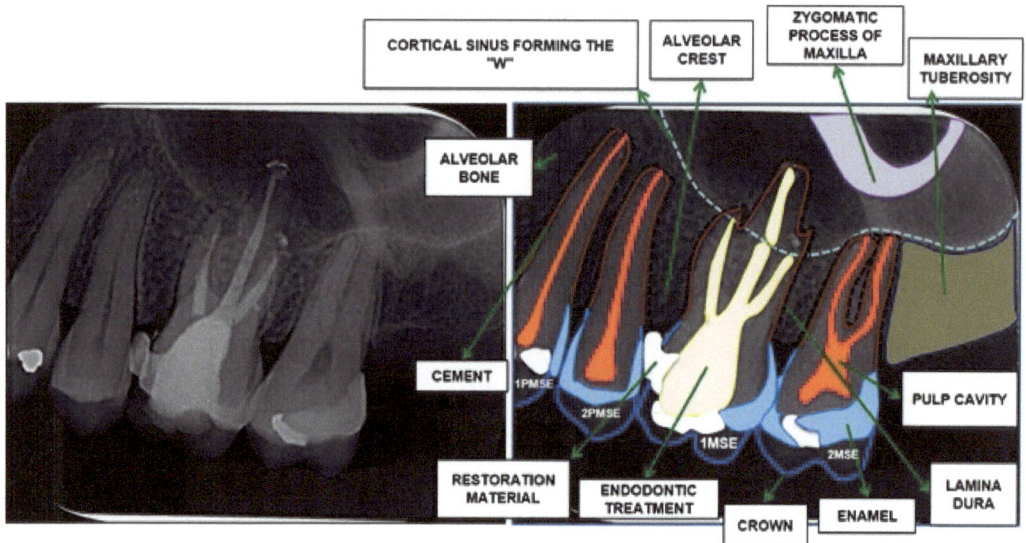

**Fig. (34).** Periapical Radiographs - Molar Region.

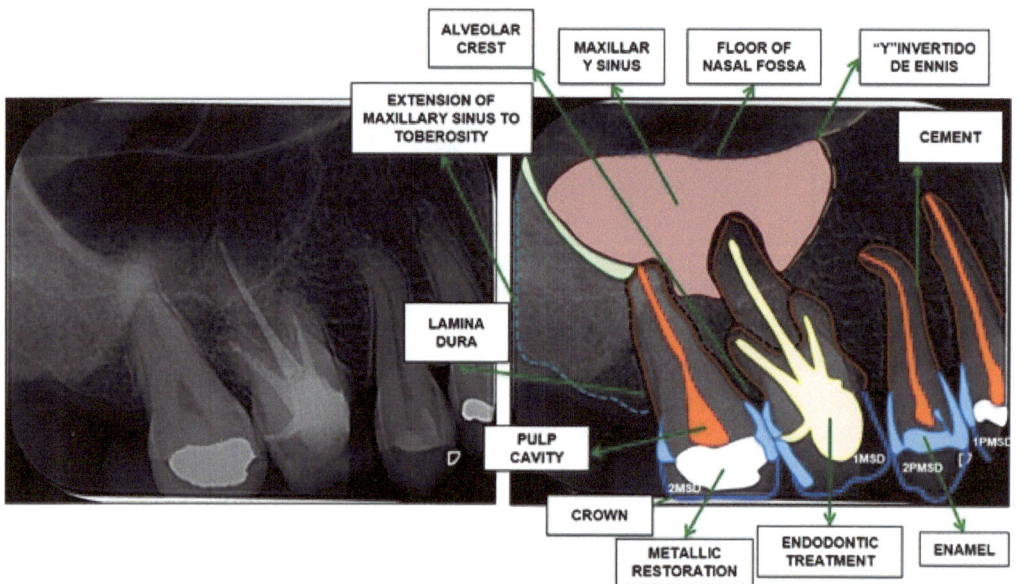

**Fig. (35).** Periapical Radiographs - Molar Region.

ZYGOMATIC PROCESS OF MAXILLA - radiographic image presents a radiopaque superimposed on region of upper molars, the shape varies with incidence of X-ray applied. It is most often observed in the form of U or V, and continues with a smaller radiopacity image and greater uniformity, corresponding to zygomatic bone (Figs. **34**, **36**).

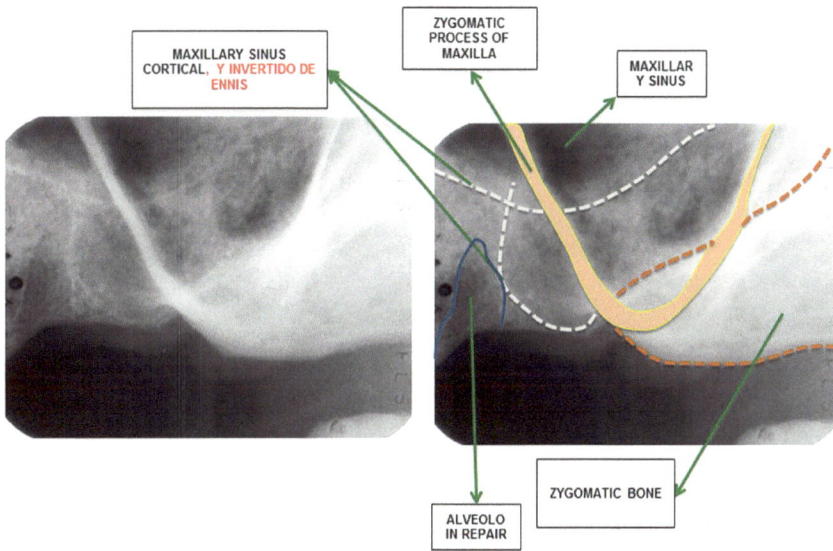

**Fig. (36).** Periapical Radiographs - Molar Region toothless.

CORONOID PROCESS - it belongs to mandible but can be seen on radiographs of the posterior maxilla. It Radiographically presents a radiopaque image, with triangular shape of sharp contours and could be below or superimposed on tuber of maxilla (Figs. **33**, **37**, **38**).

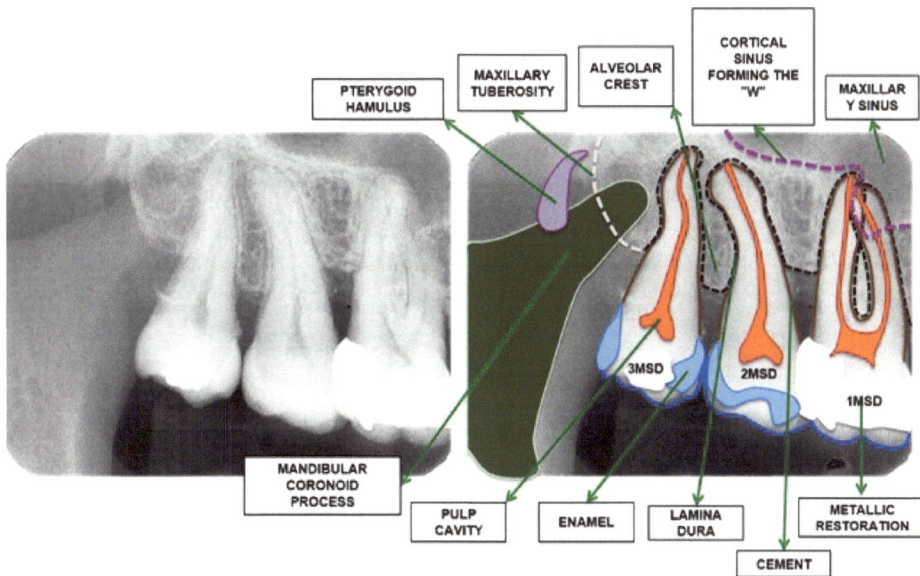

**Fig. (37).** Periapical Radiographs - Molar Region.

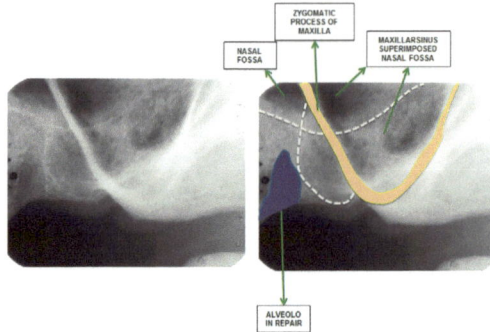

**Fig. (38).** Periapical Radiographs - Molar Region.

PTERYGOID HAMULUS - appears Radiographically as a radiopaque image. The width, shape and length are variable located at the posterior of maxilla (Figs. **32**, **37**, **43**).

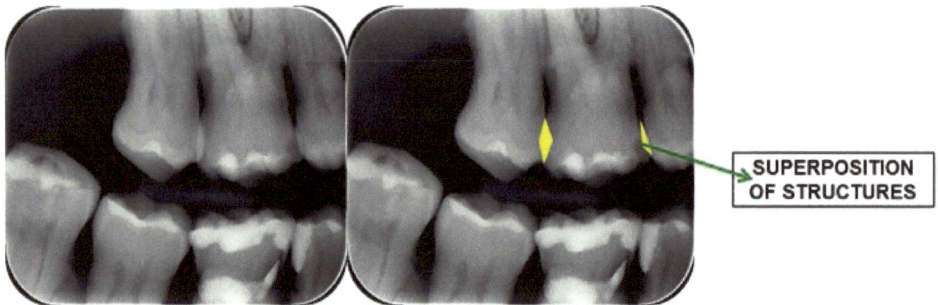

**Fig. (39).** Interproximal - Molar Region.

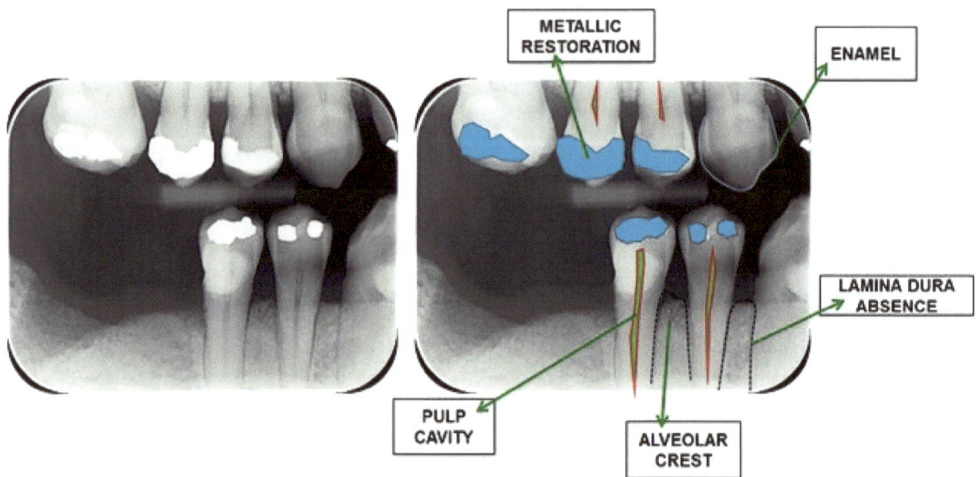

**Fig. (40).** Interproximal - Premolar Region.

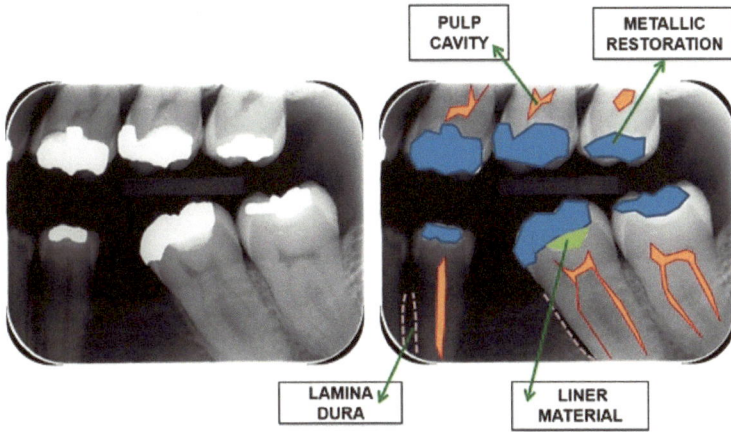

**Fig. (41).** Interproximal - Molar Region.

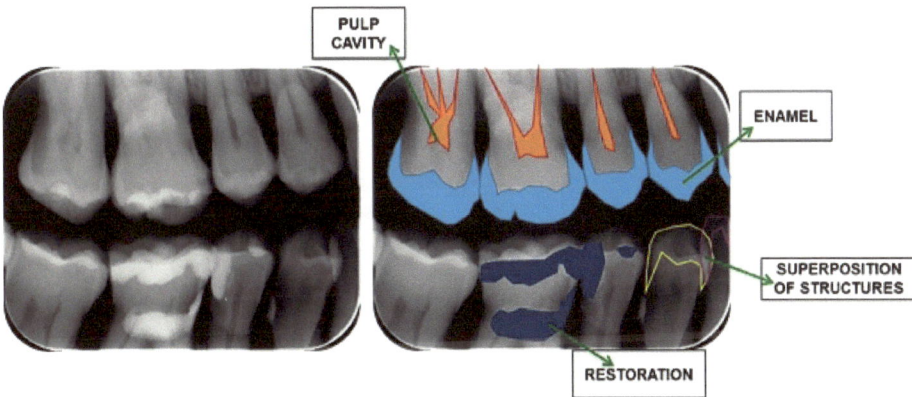

**Fig. (42).** Interproximal - Premolar and Molar Region.

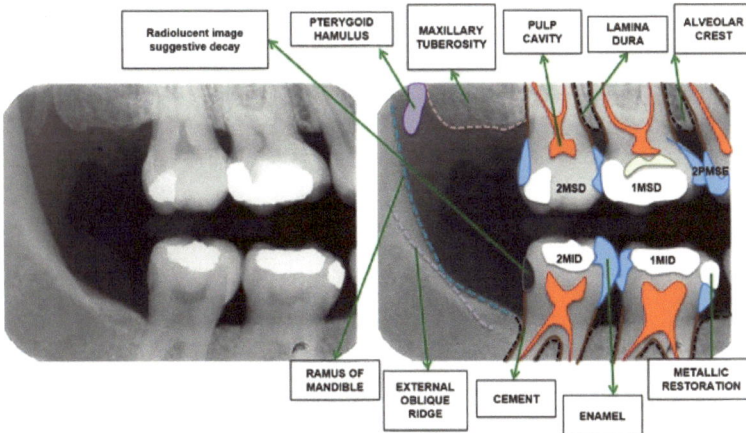

**Fig. (43).** Interproximal - Molar Region.

MAXILLARY TUBEROSITY (TUBEROSITY) - is bounded Radiographically by a radiopaque line of superior concavity which means the union of buccal and palatine cortical, located in posterior limit of the alveolar apophysis (Fig. **35**).

## Mandible Dental Regions [1 - 5]

### *Central Region*

MENTAL PROTUBERANCE - appears radiographically as an area of condensing the mandible bone, forming a radiopaque image in the incisor region with variable length, extending from the premolar region to the symphysis with pyramidal shape, the base corresponds to the lower border of mandible (Figs. **44**, **46**).

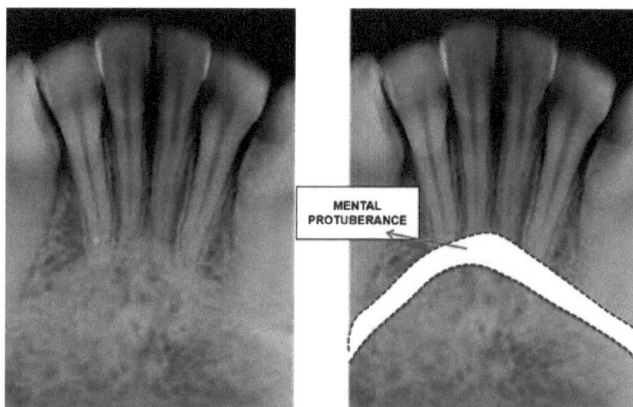

**Fig. (44).** Periapical Radiographs - CentralRegion.

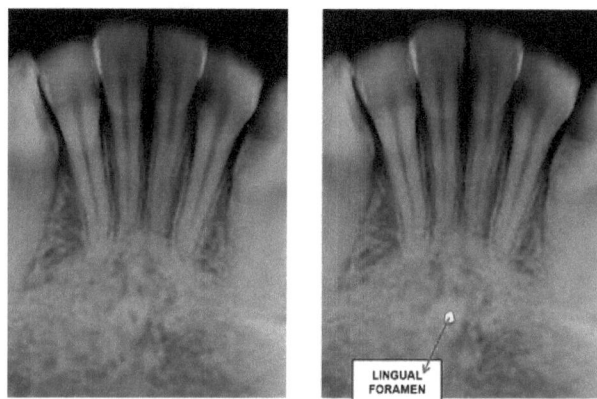

**Fig. (45).** Periapical Radiographs - CentralRegion.

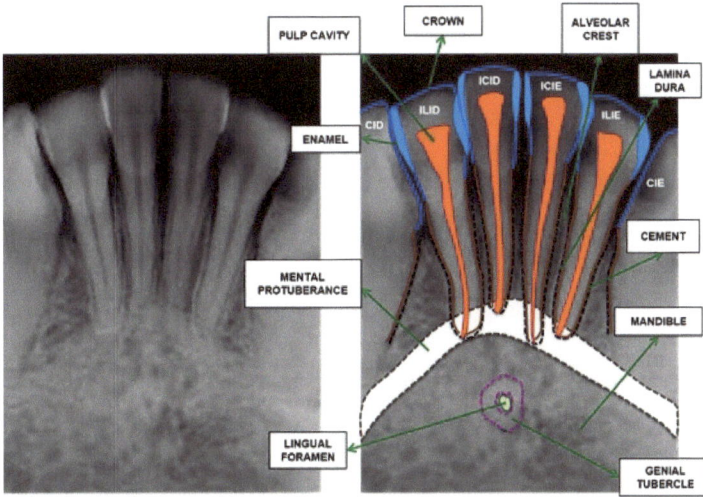

**Fig. (46).** Periapical Radiographs - CentralRegion.

LINGUAL FORAMEN - appears radiographically as a small radiolucent area, circular, located in the midline of mandible, below the apex of central incisors, usually appearing in the center of mental spine (Figs. **45**, **46**).

GENIAL TUBERCLE (MENTAL SPINE) - radiographically appears as a radiopaque ring below the apex of the central incisors, encircling the lingual foramina. Bony projections located in the midline of mandible, which gives insertion to milo-hyoid and genioglossus muscles (Fig. **47**).

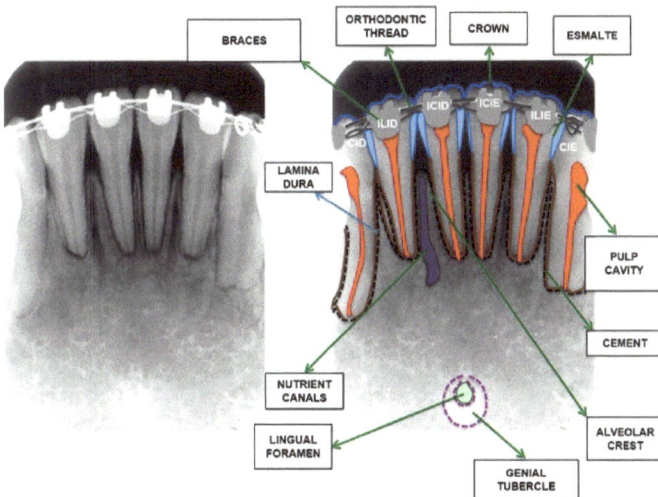

**Fig. (47).** Periapical Radiographs - CentralRegion.

NUTRIENT CANALS - is observed radiographically as radiolucent lines that correspond to the intraosseous route of arterioles or veins (Fig. **47**).

## Canine and Premolar Region (Figs. 50-52) [1 - 5]

MENTAL FORAMEN - radiographically appears as an oval or rounded radiolucent image, located in the apical region of the premolars or superimposed to them. In edentulous individuals, due to remarkable alveolar ridge resorption, its radiographic image will be located near occlusal plane (Fig. **48**).

MANDIBULAR CANAL - radiographically appears as a thick radiolucent line, delimited by radiopaque edge, below the roots of the molars and premolars, extending from the mandibular foramen to the mental foramen, passing the inferior alveolar neurovascular bundle (Fig. **49**).

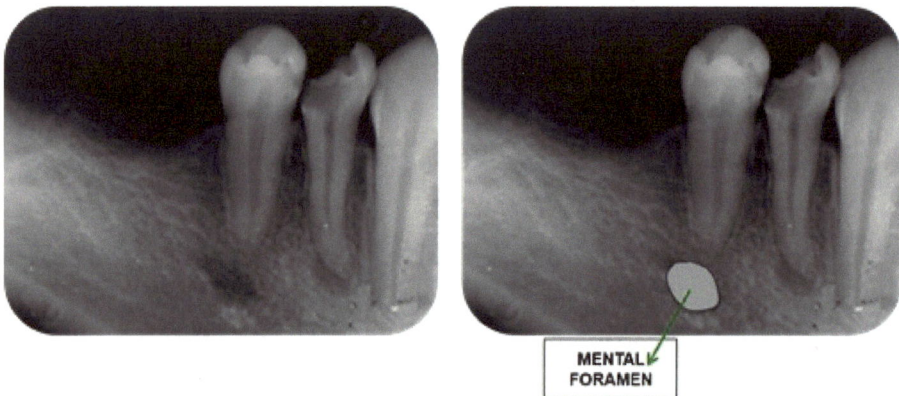

MENTAL FORAMEN

**Fig. (48).** Periapical Radiographs - Canine and Premolar Region.

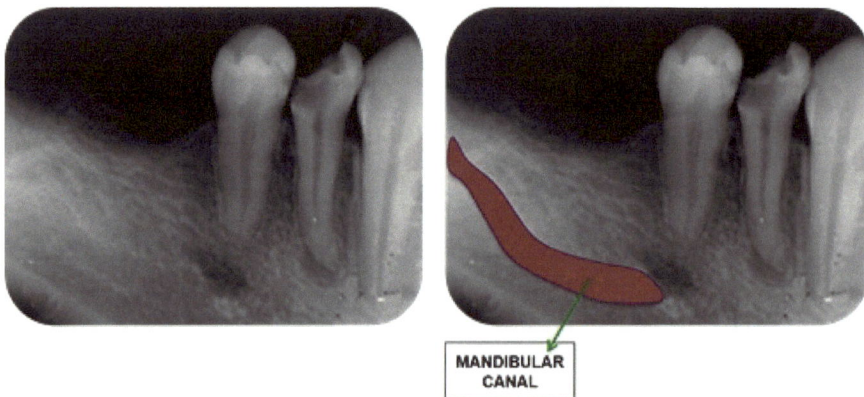

MANDIBULAR CANAL

**Fig. (49).** Periapical Radiographs - Canine and Premolar Region.

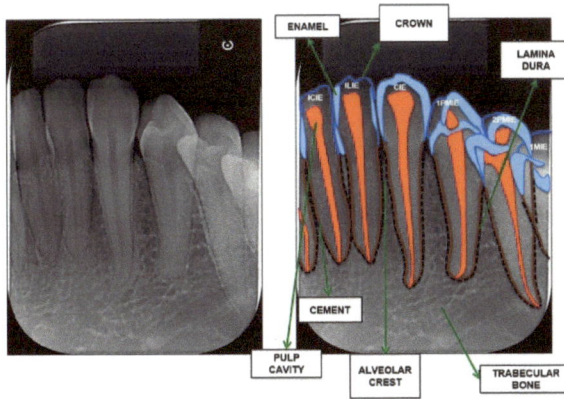

**Fig. (50).** Periapical Radiographs - Canine and Premolar Region.

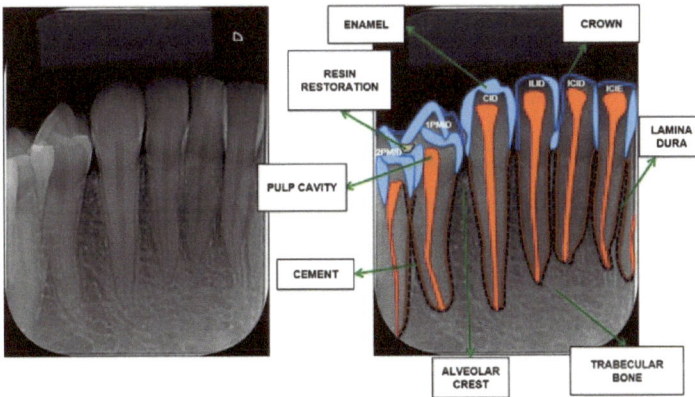

**Fig. (51).** Periapical Radiographs - Canine and Premolar Region.

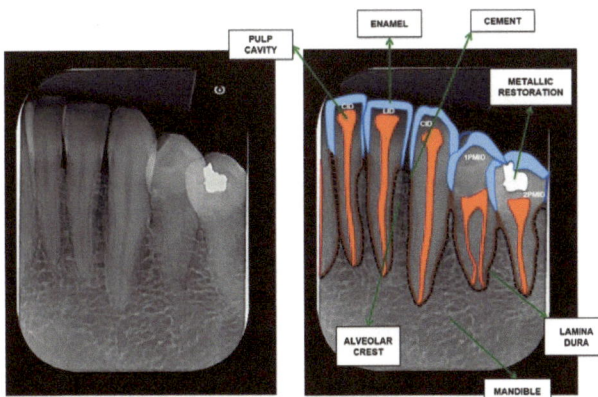

**Fig. (52).** Periapical Radiographs - Canine and Premolar Region.

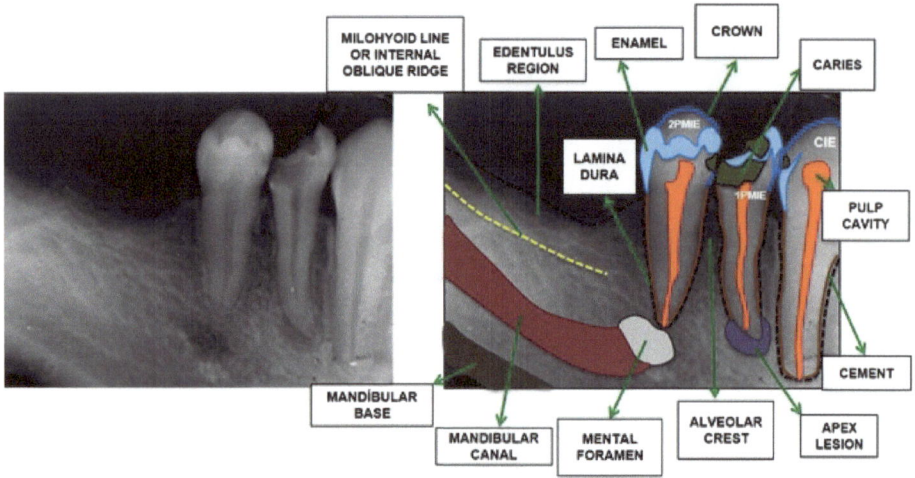

**Fig. (53).** Periapical Radiographs - Canine and Premolar Region.

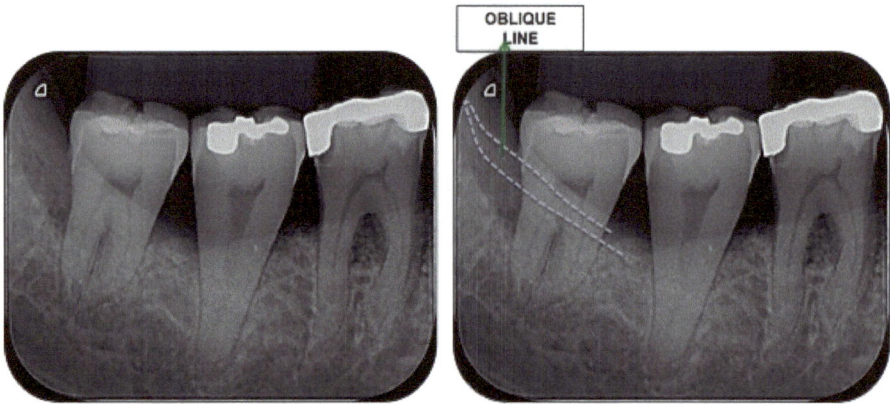

**Fig. (54).** Periapical Radiographs - Molar Region.

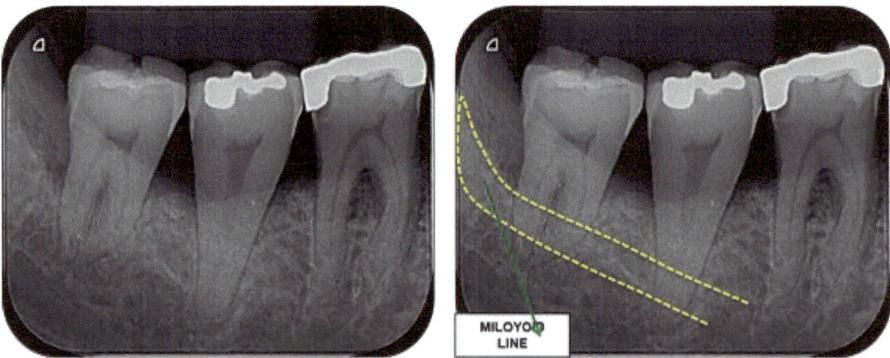

**Fig. (55).** Periapical Radiographs - Molar Region.

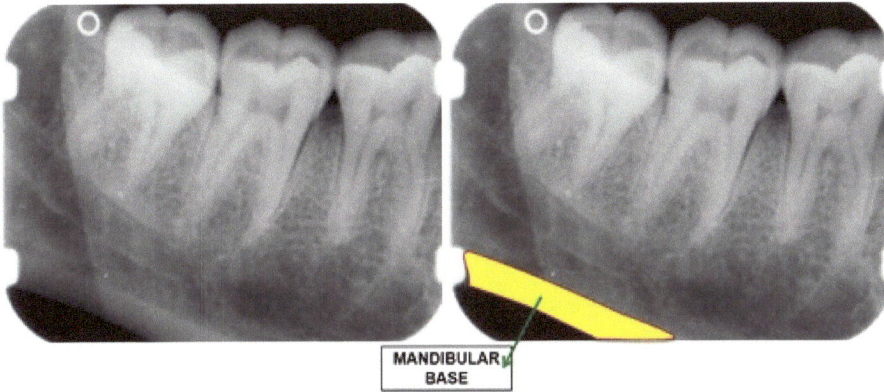

**Fig. (56).** Periapical Radiographs - Molar Region.

SUBMANDIBULAR FOSSA - radiographically, has an area of less radiopacity in the posterior mandible (Figs. **57**, **59**).

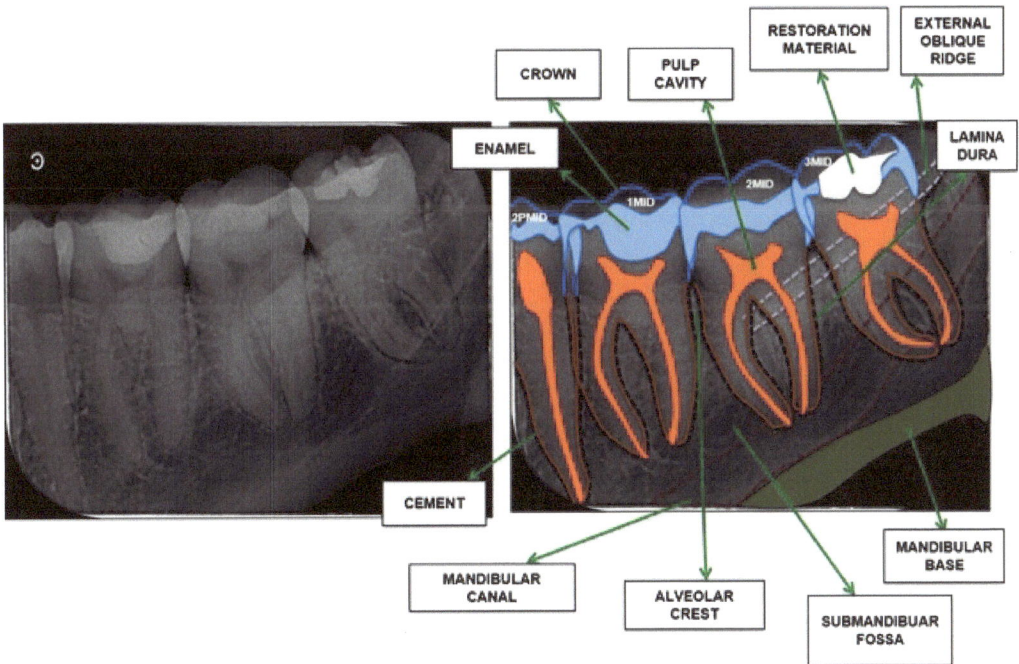

**Fig. (57).** Periapical Radiographs - Molar Region.

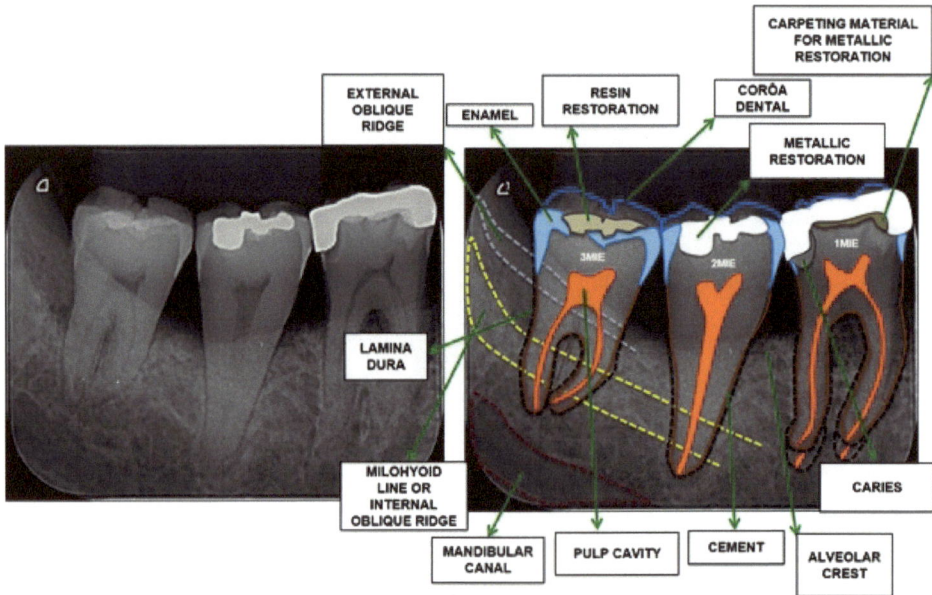

**Fig. (58).** Periapical Radiographs - Molar Region.

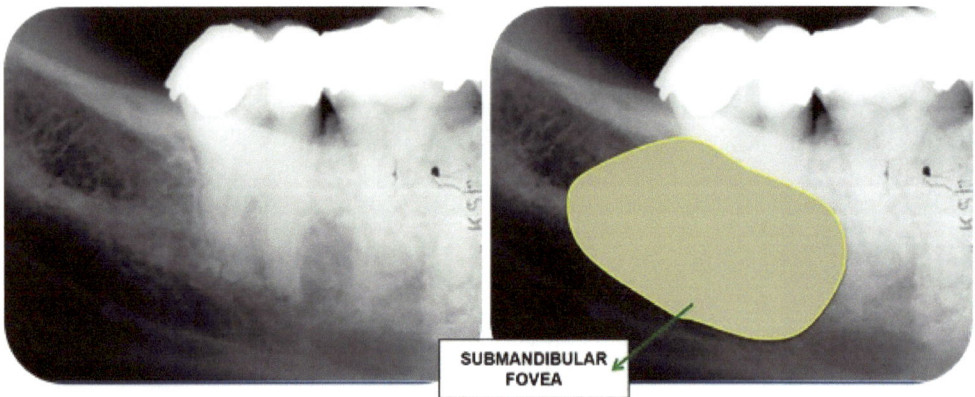

**Fig. (59).** Periapical Radiographs - Molar Region.

## Molar Region [3 - 5]

OBLIQUE RIDGE (LINE) - radiographically appears as a radiopaque line crossing transversely the mandible body to the middle of third molar roots (Figs. **53**, **54**, **56**, **58**).

MILOHIOIDEA RIDGE (LINE) - radiographically is seen as a radiopaque line originating in the middle portion of mandible branch, crossing diagonally toward the body to the level of molars (Figs. **53**, **55**, **56**, **58**).

MANDIBULAR BASE - radiographically appears as a very radiopaque line (Figs. **53**, **56**, **57**).

## Periodontium Regions [1 - 5]

The periodontium (supporting tissue) in dentistry, is the name given to all those tissues involved in teeth fixation in bone (maxilla or mandible). It Shows components with different degrees of density, thus presenting well-defined radiographically. Components: Support and Protection Periodontium.

Support periodontium is formed by the periodontal ligament, alveolar bone and cementum. Its function is to provide support, nutrition, formative and sensory effect.

CEMENT - it is not identified radiographically as a separate dentin structure, but with exceptions in cases of hyperplasia, it becomes thicker than normal (Figs. **61-64**).

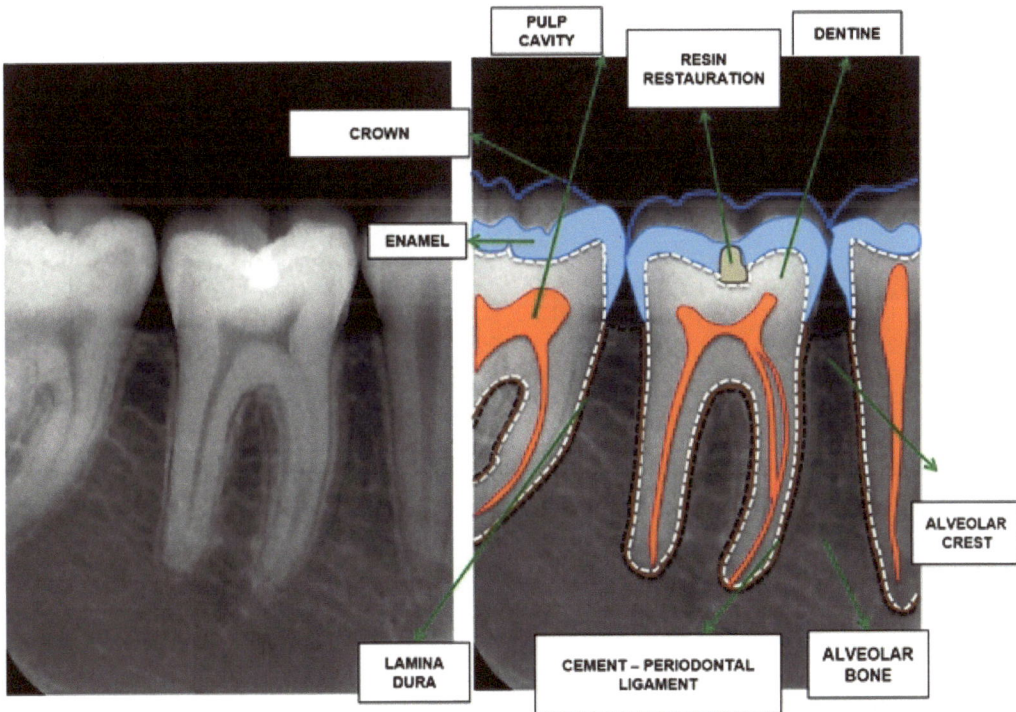

**Fig. (60).** Periapical Radiographs - Periodontium.

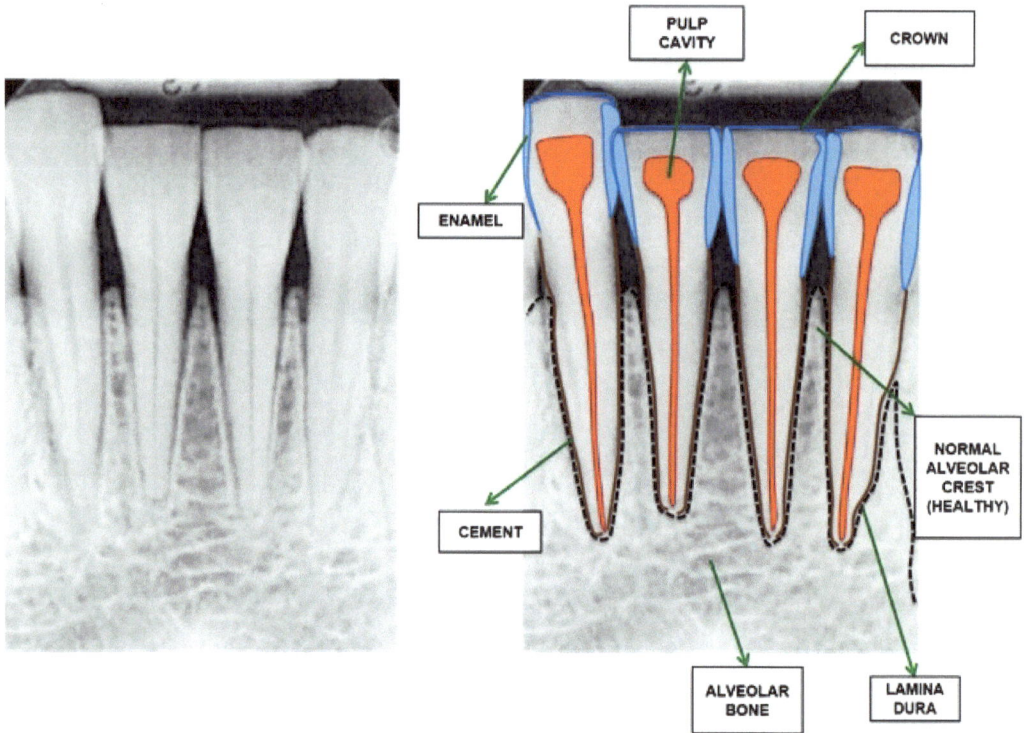

**Fig. (61).** Periapical Radiographs - Normal Periodontium - Anterior Mandibular Region.

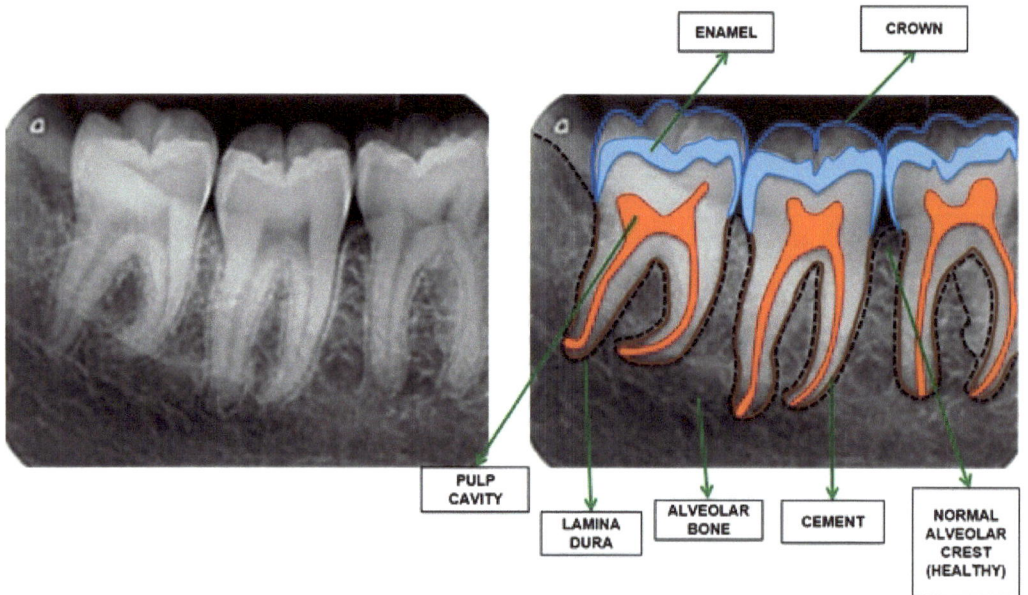

**Fig. (62).** Periapical Radiographs - Normal Periodontium - Posteiror Mandibular Region.

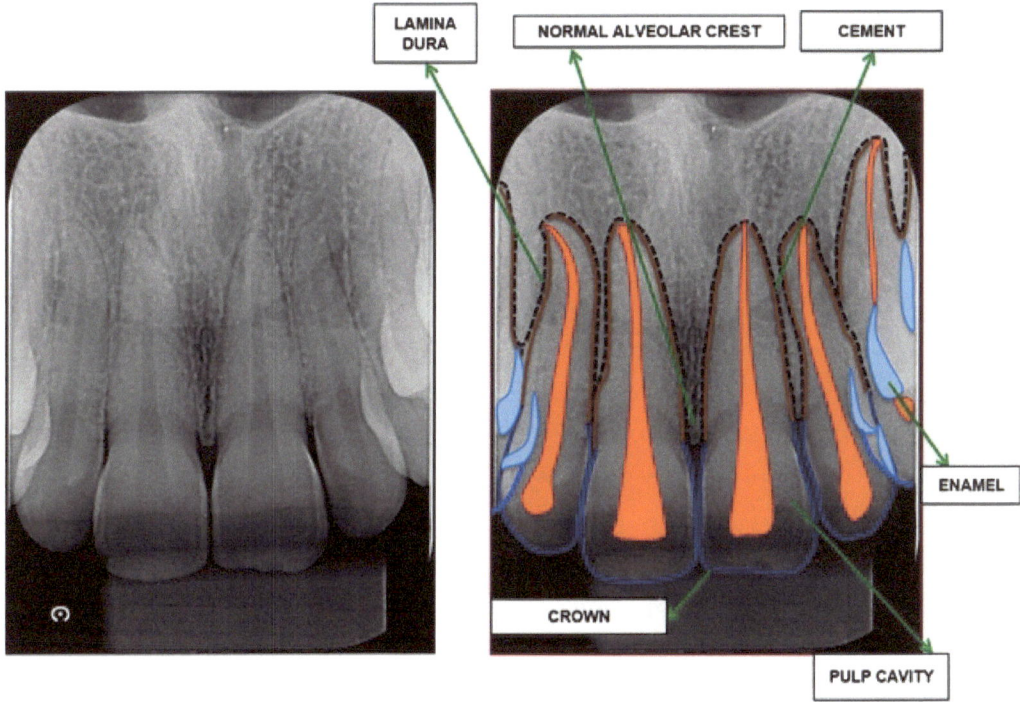

**Fig. (63).** Periapical Radiographs - Normal Periodontium - Anterior Maxillary Region.

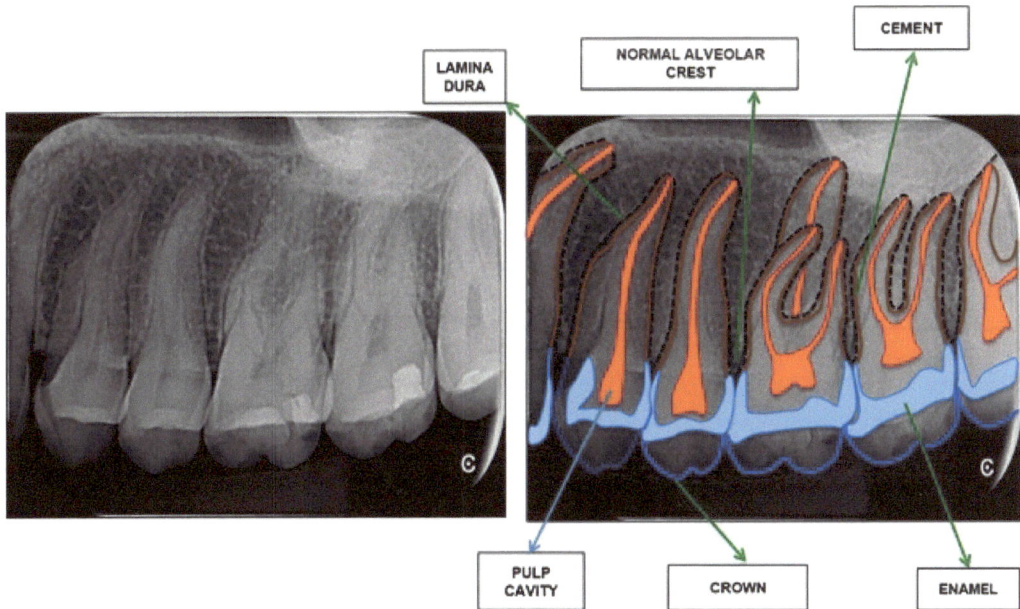

**Fig. (64).** Periapical Radiographs - Normal Periodontium - Posterior Maxilla Region.

PERIODONTAL LIGAMENT - it is the system that connects tooth to the bone and forms by dense modeled conjunctive tissue. In the bone, it presents a syndesmosis joint type, showing two resistant tissues permeated by fibers (stretch and contraction), having an average thickness of 0.2 mm (0.1 to 0.4 mm). It is responsible for bone and cementum union and performs the damping forces (oblique fibers and tissue fluid), bone and root remodeling, sensory (presence of proprioceptors) and nutritious (blood supply). It consists of 5 types of collagen fibers divided into: alveolar crest fibers, horizontal fibers, interradicular fibers, oblique fibers (in higher proportion) and apical fibers. The periodontal ligament is essential for tooth mobility (Fig. **60**).

ALVEOLAR BONE - It is the portion of the jaws that form and support the tooth sockets and is developed in association with the development and eruption tooth. Bone can be divided in to compact bone (alveolar bone, also called lamina dura, lining the sockets and has canals that passes blood vessels, lymphatics and nerve fibers to the periodontal ligament) and the spongy bone (fills the areas between the dental socket and compact bone walls, occupying most of the interdental septum forming bone trabeculae). It is identified with radiographic appearance of a trabecular structure, radiopaque, radiotransparent medullary delimiting areas where this architectural distribution, the shape and size of their trabeculae, are directly linked to forces acting on jaws. Importantly, as a result, with time physiological changes the trabecular bone.

LAMINA DURA OR ALVEOLAR CORTICAL - it is identified radiographically as a radiopaque line, uniform, suffering variations as the morphology of the tooth root, is the wall of the socket where the periodontal fibers are inserted and continue to be uninterrupted to form ALVEOLAR CREST where the periodontal disease can be studied. Functions of alveolar bone - Support for dental elements, nutrition, absorption and distribution of forces and regulation of chewing movements (Fig. **60**).

LIGAMENT+BONE+CEMENT = dental insertion apparatus

Protection periodontium formed by the gingiva (marginal, interdental and attached gingiva). Gingiva is fixed, inserted into bone, has no mobility. The gingiva is part of the masticatory mucosa covering the alveolar process and surrounds the cervical portion of tooth. Consists of an epithelial layer and an underlying connective tissue called the lamina propria (Figs. **60**, **63**, **64**).

KERATINIZED MUCOSA - Varies 1-9 mm probing depth. Clinical importance is the immobilization of gingival margin and sealing between internal environment and the external environment.

GINGIVAL SULCUS - Depth varies from 0.5 - 1.0 mm and its amplitude varies from 0.15 - 0.25 mm. Clinically it is considered normal when there is no bleeding on probing and one is considered sick when bleeding occurs on probing.

JUNCTIONAL EPITHELIUM - Promotes the contact of the gingiva with the tooth, presents a probing of 0.9 to 1.3mm. It has a high index of renewal that occurs in the basal layer (mitoses in the basal layer, renew all epithelia, but the junctional is renewed more). It is not a keratinized tissue. Clinically it allows the penetration of the probe to the beginning of the connection with the connective tissue.

## Horizontal and Vertical Bone Loss [1 - 5]

Vertical and horizontal bone resorption of the alveolar bone (periodontal lesions) include those conditions that primarily involve the periodontal tissues. These consist of gingiva, periodontal ligament and alveolar bone. There are different indexes used to reveal the stage of periodontal disease, which are often based on the measurement using the radiographs and radiographic aspects (Fig. **65**).

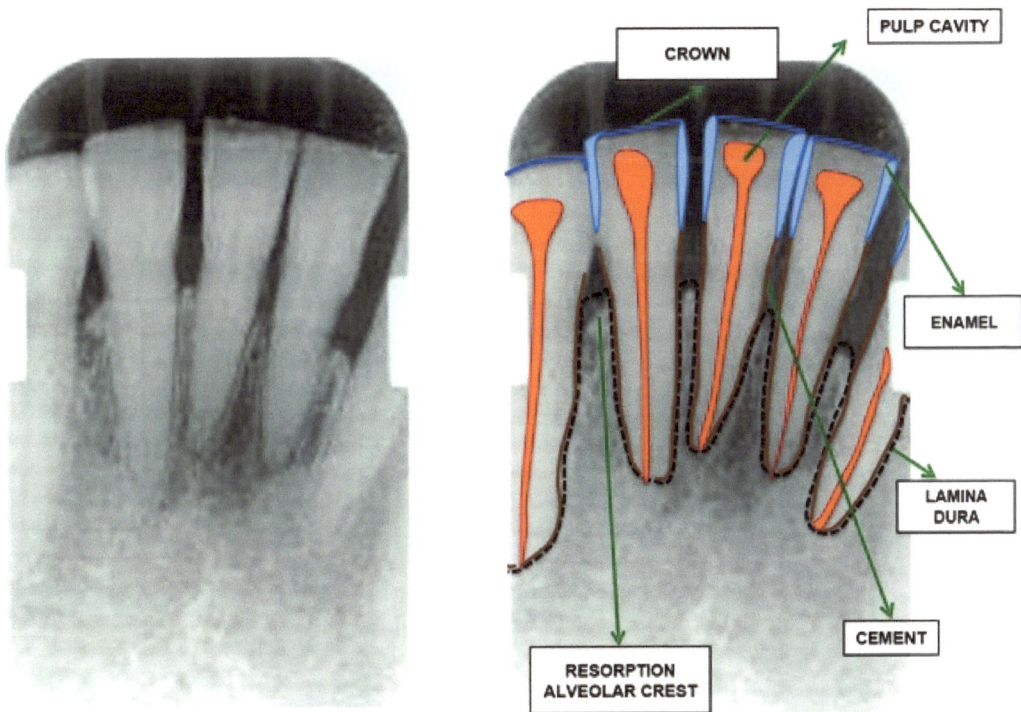

**Fig. (65).** Periapical Radiographs - Horizontal Bone Loss - Anterior Mandibular Region.

HORIZONTAL BONE LOSS - caused by the extension of gingival inflammation is responsible for the reduction in height of the alveolar bone, occurs when bone loss is parallel to cementoenamel junction (CE), 1 to 1.5 mm below the CE. Radiographically observed loss of cortical alveolar crest, radiolucent image in the central portion of crest and occurs the reduction of "physiological level" below 1-1.5 mm from CE with a decrease in height of alveolar crest (Figs. **66-68**).

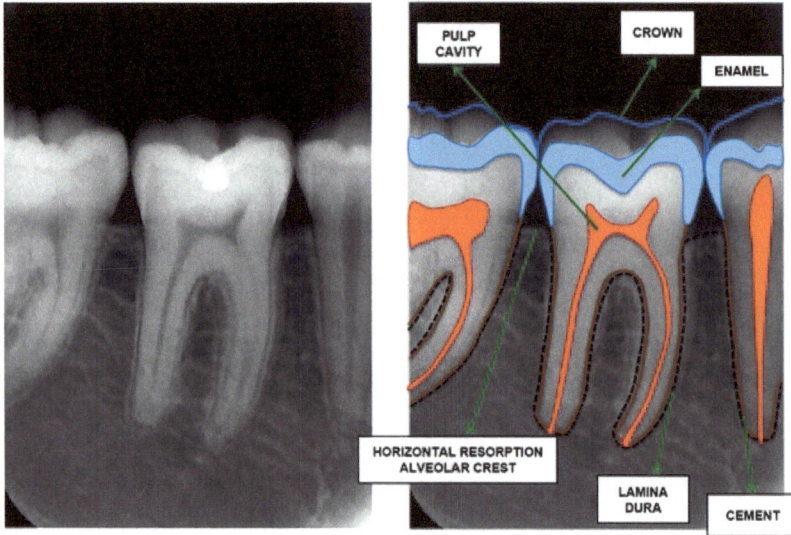

**Fig. (66).** Periapical Radiographs - Horizontal Bone Loss - Posterior Mandibular Region.

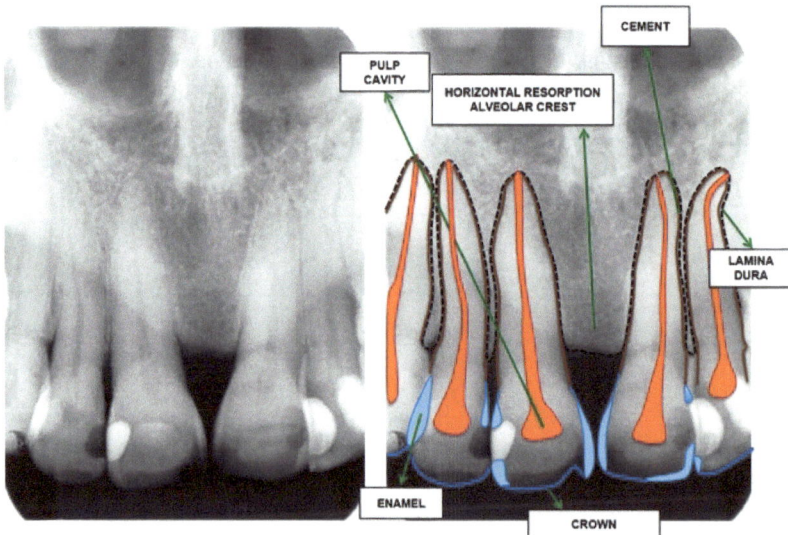

**Fig. (67).** Periapical Radiographs - Horizontal Bone Loss - Anterior Maxilla Region.

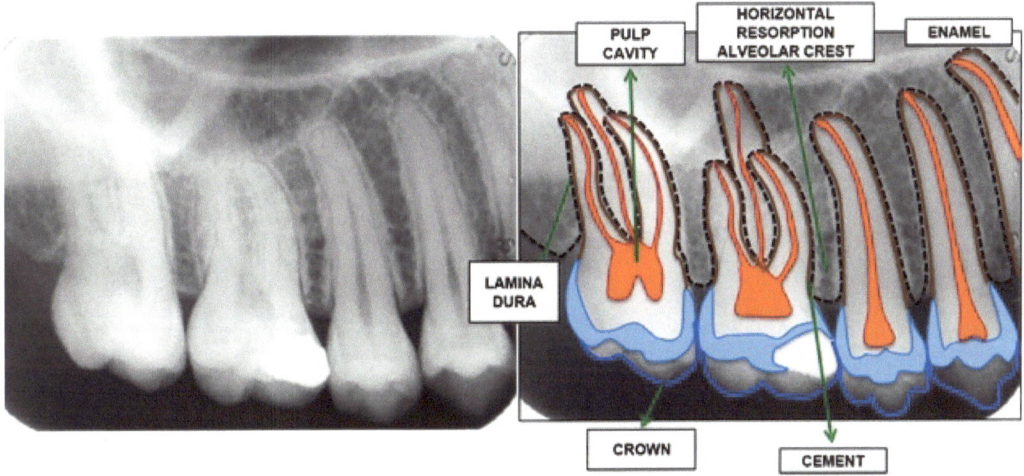

**Fig. (68).** Periapical Radiographs - Horizontal Bone Loss - Posterior Maxilla Region.

VERTICAL BONE LOSS - occurs mainly by occlusion trauma leading to laterally bone loss to the root surface, occurring in angular direction, oblique, starting on the side portion of alveolar crest due to progression of inflammation or due to occlusal trauma. During the horizontal bone loss, vertical loss can occur, since the trauma acts with inflammatory reactions (Figs. **69-72**).

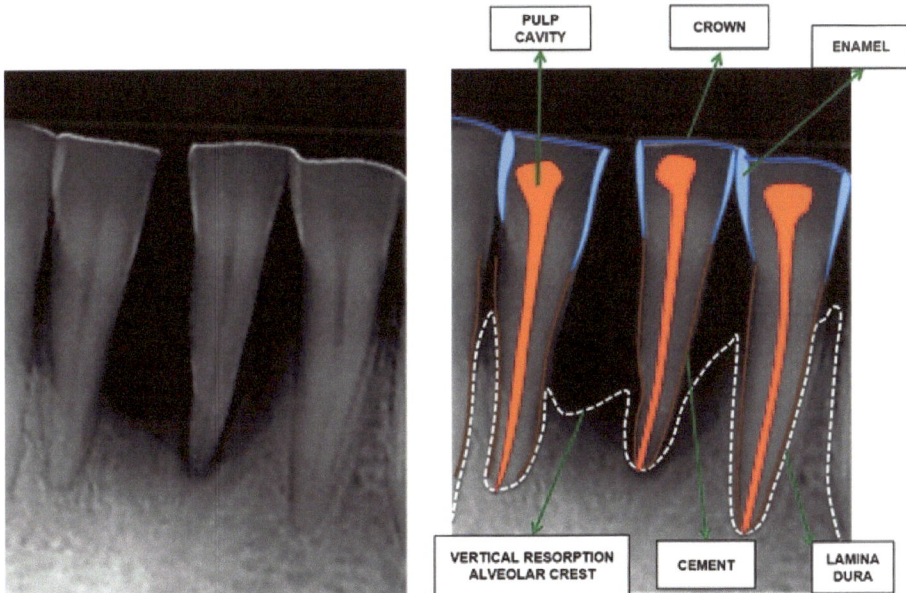

**Fig. (69).** Periapical Radiographs - Vertical Bone Loss - Anterior Mandibular Region.

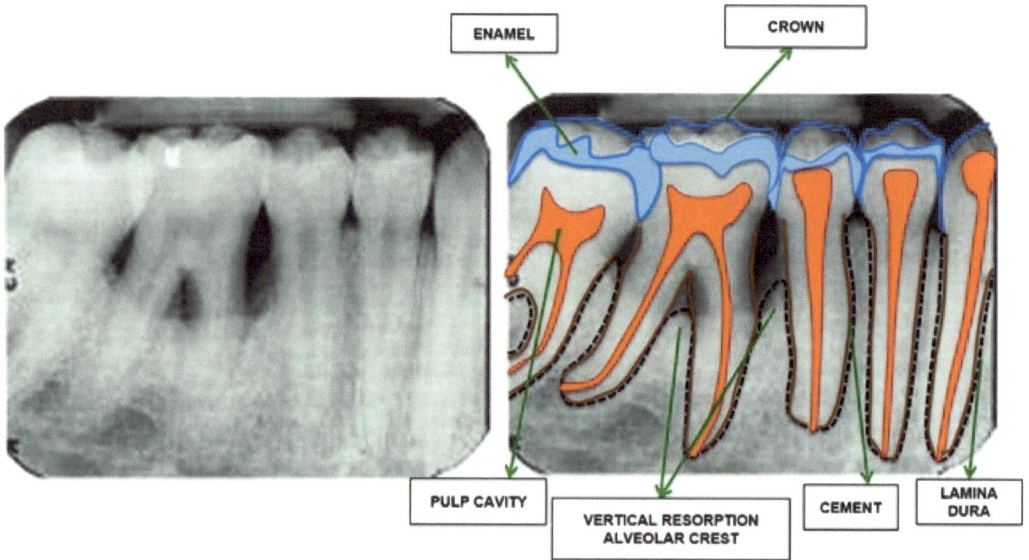

**Fig. (70).** Periapical Radiographs - Vertical Bone Loss - Posterior Mandibular Region.

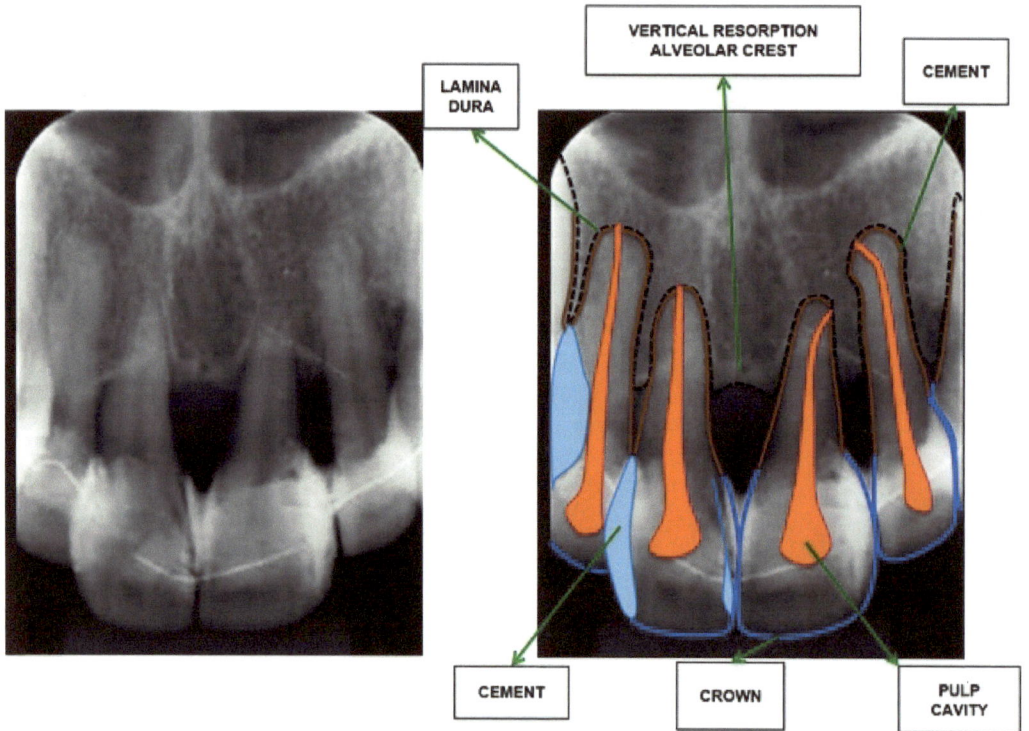

**Fig. (71).** Periapical Radiographs - Vertical Bone Loss - Anterior Maxilla Region.

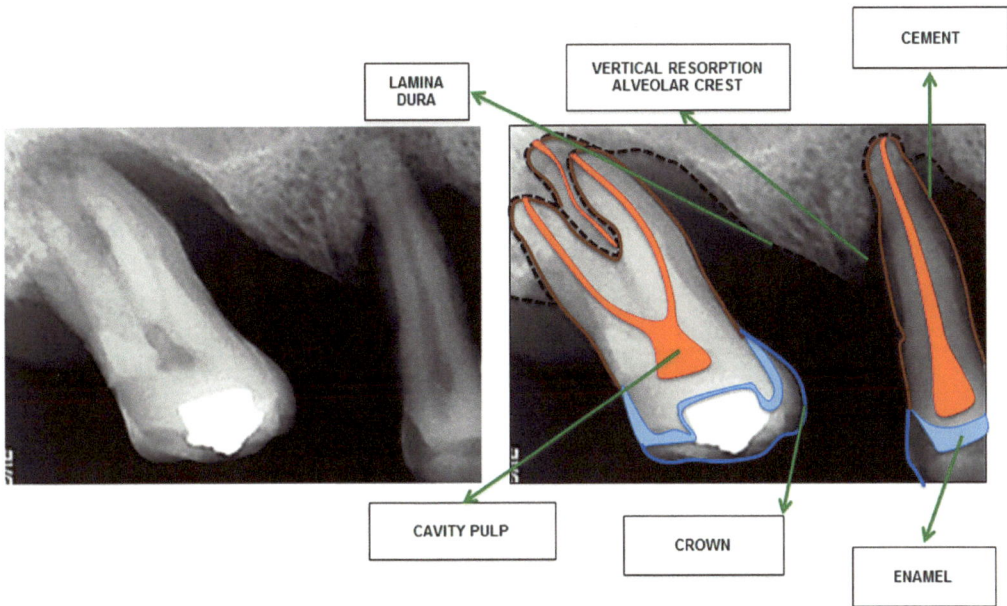

**Fig. (72).** Periapical Radiographs - Vertical Bone Loss - Posterior Maxilla Region.

## Furcation Involvement [3 - 5]

FURCATION is a unique anatomical feature of multirooted teeth: being defined as the area between the roots where they begin to separate below the cervical portion. When periodontal disease affects this level, there is the furcation involvement or lesion, characterized by bone resorption and insertion loss in interradicular space (Fig. **73**).

GRADES indices vary according to the involvement of the furcation: GRADE 1 - is considered the initial or early stage of the lesion which does not show noticeable changes in radiography. GRADE 2 - it is the increased horizontal component and can affect one or more forces on the same tooth. GRADE 3, is the furcation of lesions that can be visualized radiographically and inter-radicular bone loss. GRADE 4 - destroyed inter-radicular bone and soft tissue retraction, since lesion exists in the bone wall that holds tooth, gingiva recession and other soft tissues.

Predisposing factors (leading to occur furcation lesion), anatomy or natural morphology root and furcation size, accessories canals, caused by a bone defect, periodontitis or decay, occlusal trauma and iatrogenic factors.

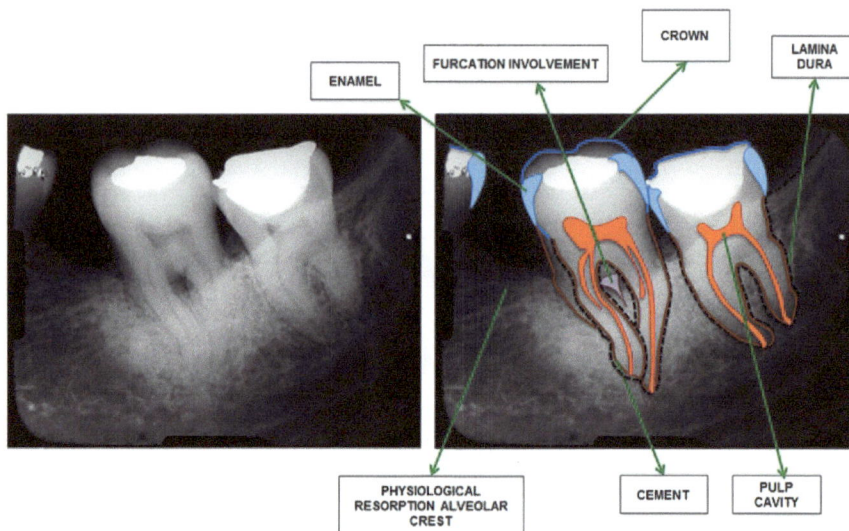

**Fig. (73).** Periapical Radiographs - Furcation Involvement.

## Occlusal Radiographs [4 - 5]

Occlusal radiography is an additional radiographic examination designed to provide a broader view of the maxilla and mandible. The occlusal radiography is very useful to determine the buccal-lingual expansion of pathological conditions such as cysts and tumors, and provides additional information about the extent and the displacement of the jaws fractures. Occlusal films also help the location of impacted teeth, residual roots, foreign bodies, and calculus in the submandibular and sublingual salivary glands and ducts. It should be noted when evaluating soft tissues, the exposure time needs to be appropriately reduced (Figs. **74-78**).

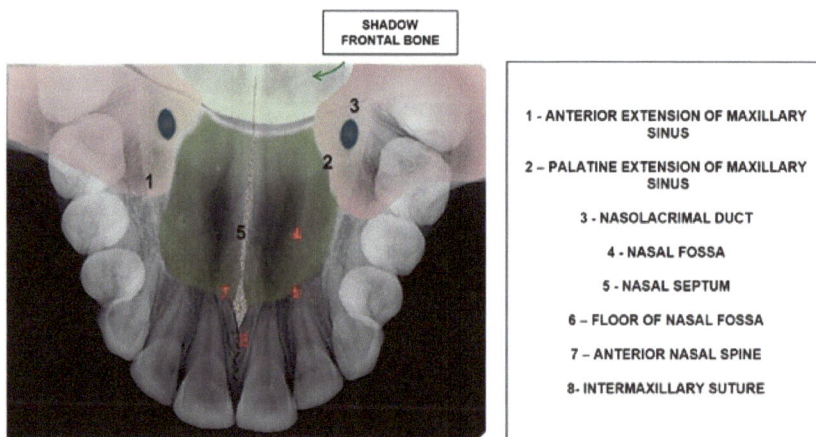

**Fig. (74).** Maxillary Occlusal Technique.

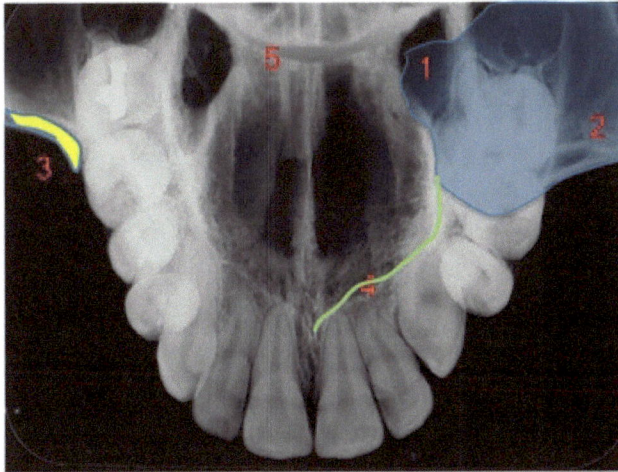

1 - PALATINE EXTENSION BETWEEN PALATINE PROCESS CORTICAL

2 – ZYGOMATIC EXTENSION AND ZYGOMATIC PROCESS

3 - ZYGOMATIC PROCESS

4 - FLOOR OF NASAL FOSSA

5 - SHADOW FRONTAL BONE

**Fig. (75).** Maxillary Occlusal Technique.

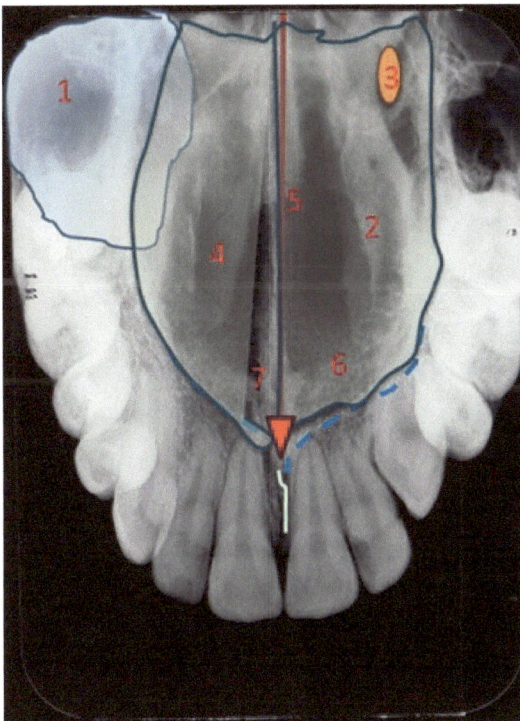

1 – PALATINE EXTENSION OF MAXILLARY SINUS

2 - ANTERIOR EXTENSION OF MAXILLARY SINUS

3 - NASOLACRIMAL DUCT

4 - NASAL FOSSA

5 - NASAL SEPTUM

6 – FLOOR OF NASAL FOSSA

7 – ANTERIOR NASAL SPINE

**Fig. (76).** Maxillary Occlusal Technique.

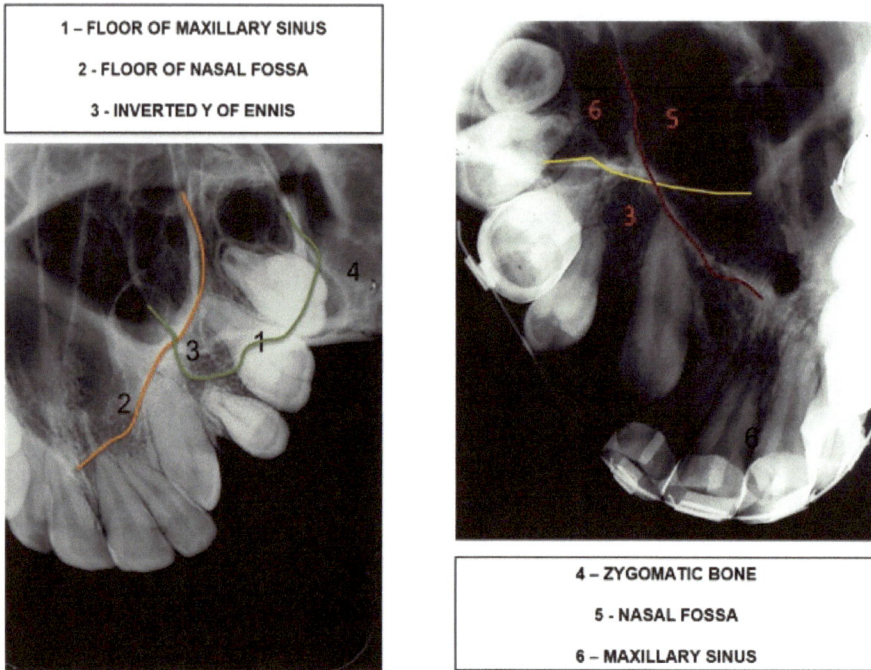

1 – FLOOR OF MAXILLARY SINUS

2 - FLOOR OF NASAL FOSSA

3 - INVERTED Y OF ENNIS

4 – ZYGOMATIC BONE

5 - NASAL FOSSA

6 – MAXILLARY SINUS

**Fig. (77).** Upper Canine Occlusal.

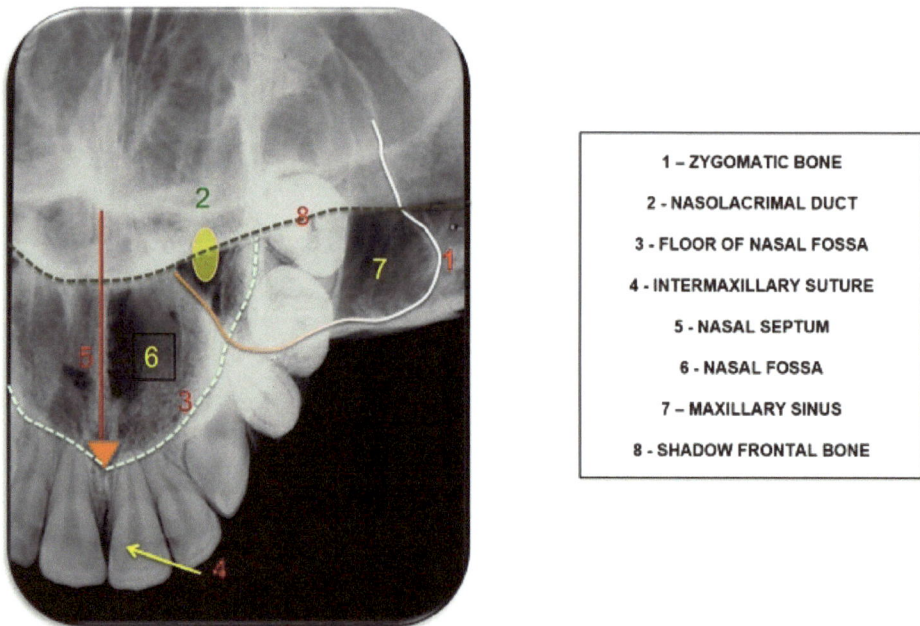

1 – ZYGOMATIC BONE

2 - NASOLACRIMAL DUCT

3 - FLOOR OF NASAL FOSSA

4 - INTERMAXILLARY SUTURE

5 - NASAL SEPTUM

6 - NASAL FOSSA

7 – MAXILLARY SINUS

8 - SHADOW FRONTAL BONE

**Fig. (78).** Upper Canine Occlusal.

## Mandibular Occlusal Technique

Mentual protuberance is an anatomical repair characterized by condensation bone of the labial surface and can also be observed in periapical radiographs of lower incisors.

Two mental spines protrude from the internal surface (5) which attach to genioglossus and genius-hioideo tendons. Above located lingual foramina, crossed by a branch of the nerve incisive and lingual artery (Figs. **79-81**).

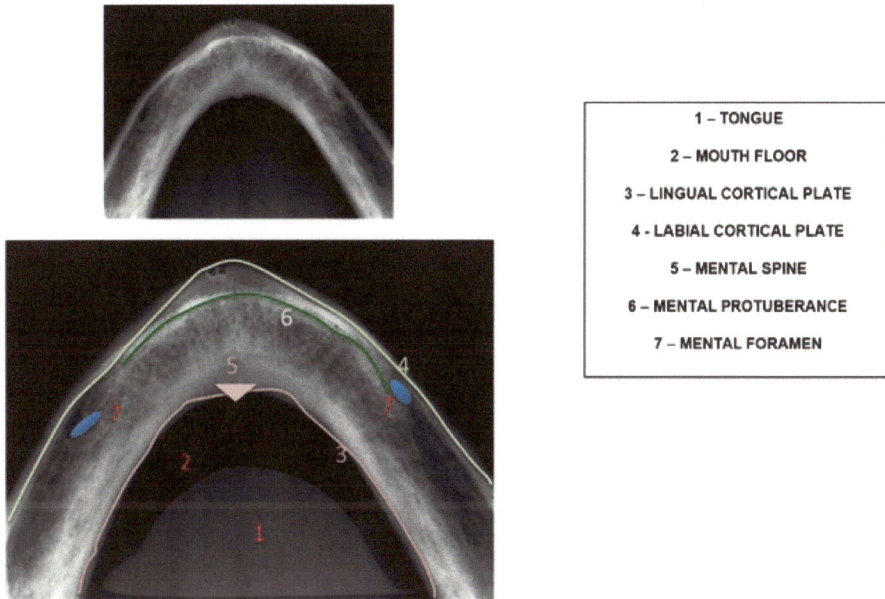

1 – TONGUE

2 – MOUTH FLOOR

3 – LINGUAL CORTICAL PLATE

4 - LABIAL CORTICAL PLATE

5 – MENTAL SPINE

6 – MENTAL PROTUBERANCE

7 – MENTAL FORAMEN

**Fig. (79).** Mandibular Occlusal Technique.

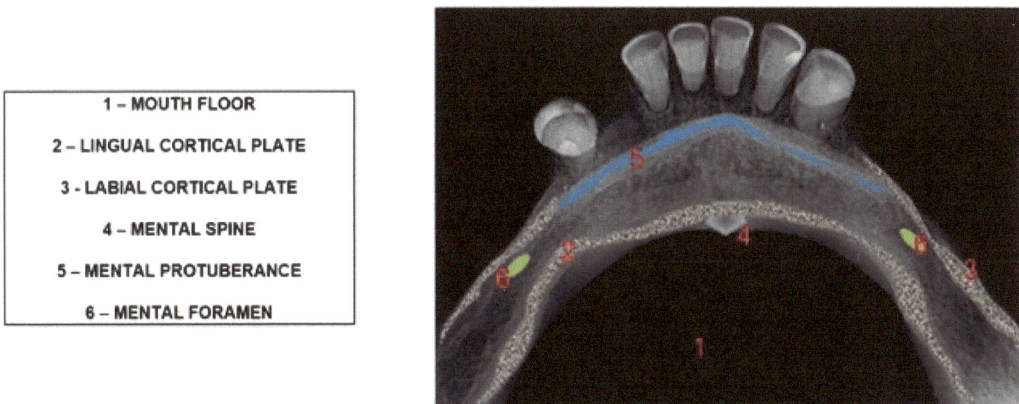

1 – MOUTH FLOOR

2 – LINGUAL CORTICAL PLATE

3 - LABIAL CORTICAL PLATE

4 – MENTAL SPINE

5 – MENTAL PROTUBERANCE

6 – MENTAL FORAMEN

**Fig. (80).** Mandibular Occlusal Technique.

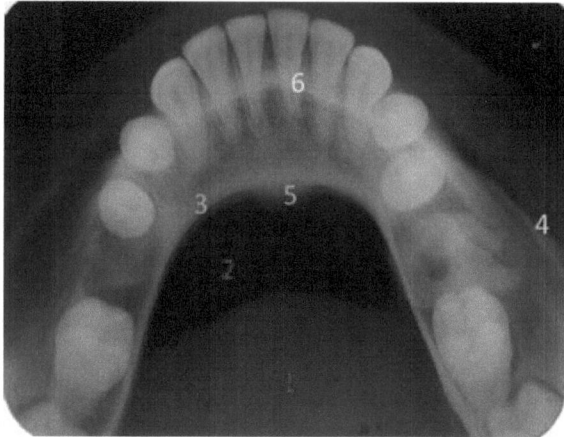

| 1 – TONGUE |
| 2 – MOUTH FLOOR |
| 3 – LINGUAL CORTICAL PLATE |
| 4 - LABIAL CORTICAL PLATE |
| 5 – MENTAL SPINE |
| 6 – MENTAL PROTUBERANCE |

**Fig. (81).** Mandibular Occlusal Technique.

## CONCLUSION

Intraoral techniques provide the highest accuracy for detailed interpretation of dental tissues and surrounding structures, including anomalies and pathologies. Use low doses of radiation to the patient and should whenever possible be performed with electronic film / sensor positioning devices, observing the principle of ALADA radioprotection ("as low as diagnostically acceptable").

## CONSENT FOR PUBLICATION

Not applicable.

## CONFLICT OF INTEREST

Radiographic material of the NACEDO - Nucleus of Support to Culture and Extension in Dental Diagnosis of the Pro-Rectory of Culture and University Extension (PRCExU / USP). Crowded at the School of Dentistry of Ribeirão Preto / University of São Paulo.

## ACKNOWLEDGEMENTS

NACEDO-PRCExU/USP

## REFERENCES

[1]    Borghetti RL, Nora VP, Costa Filho LC, Morosolli AR. Rockenbach. Projection of the oblique line in periapical radiographs of mandibular molars. Rev Odonto Ciênc 2010; 25(4): 401-5.

[2]    Freitas A, Rosa JE, Souza IF. Odontologic Radiographic. 6th ed., São Paulo: Artes Médicas 2004.

[3]    Madeira MC. Face Anatomy. 7th ed., São Paulo: Sarvier 2010.

[4]    Watanabe PC, Arita ES. Radiologia Odontológica e Imaginologia. 1st ed., Rio de Janeiro: Elsevier

2012.

[5]    White SC, Pharoah MJ. Oral Radiology - Principles and Interpretation. 7th ed., Rio de Janeiro: Elsevier 2015.

# CHAPTER 4

# Anatomy of Extraoral Techniques

**Plauto C. A. Watanabe**[*]**, Emiko S. Arita, Angela J. Camargo** and **Marina G. Baladi**

*School of Dentistry of Ribeirão Preto, University of São Paulo, São Paulo, Brazil*

**Abstract:** The radiographic image must be recorded appropriately to aid in the organization of the thoughts of the one who interprets the image and so that it may be useful for other purposes. In order to evaluate the pathological condition, the radiographic image of the normal anatomical structure must be correctly known. The extraoral techniques allow to cover a larger area of the maxillo-mandibular complex, mainly allowing to evaluate the extension of certain pathologies, and the comparison between the sides of the patient.

**Keywords:** Axial, Cephalometric Lateral, Cranial, Maxillo-mandibular complex, Panoramic radiography, Postero-anterior, TMJ.

## CRANIAL [1 - 4]

It is mainly receptacle for the most highly developed of the nervous system, brain and sensory organs involving the initial part of the digestive and respiratory systems; systems which communicate with the external environment.

The skull is divided into two parts: the neurocranium and viscerocranium. The neurocranium consists of eight bones, two temporals, two parietals, one frontal, one occipital, one sphenoid and one ethmoid. The viscerocranium is made up of 14 bones, two jaws, two palatines, two zygomatic, two lacrimal, two nasals, two inferior nasal conchae, one vomer and one mandible (Figs. **1-7**).

## Cross Section of Skull [1 - 4]

The interior view of the skull allowed to observe the edges (cortical and diploe) and the basilar region that is very rich in anatomical accidents and is divided into three fossa in different levels. The anterior cranial fossa uppermost level, middle cranial fossa (sphenoid and temporal) and posterior cranial fossa (Figs. **8-12**).

---

[*] **Corresponding author Plauto C. A. Watanabe:** School of Dentistry of Ribeirão Preto, University of São Paulo, São Paulo, Brazil; Tel: 55-16-33153993; E-mail: watanabe@forp.usp.br

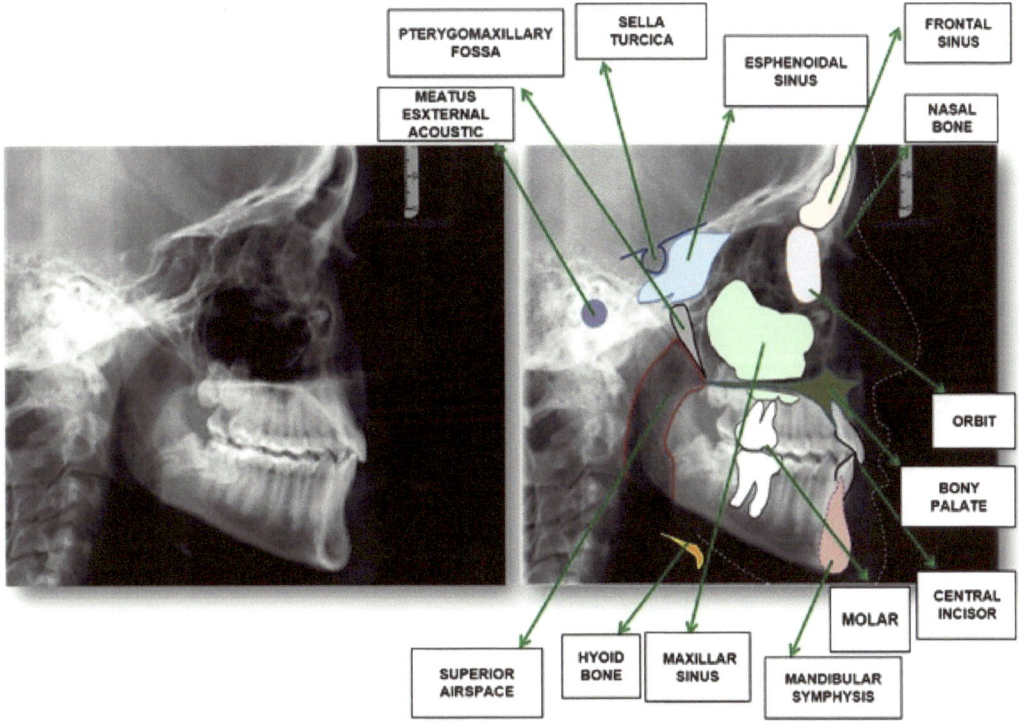

**Fig. (1).** Cephalometric Radiography.

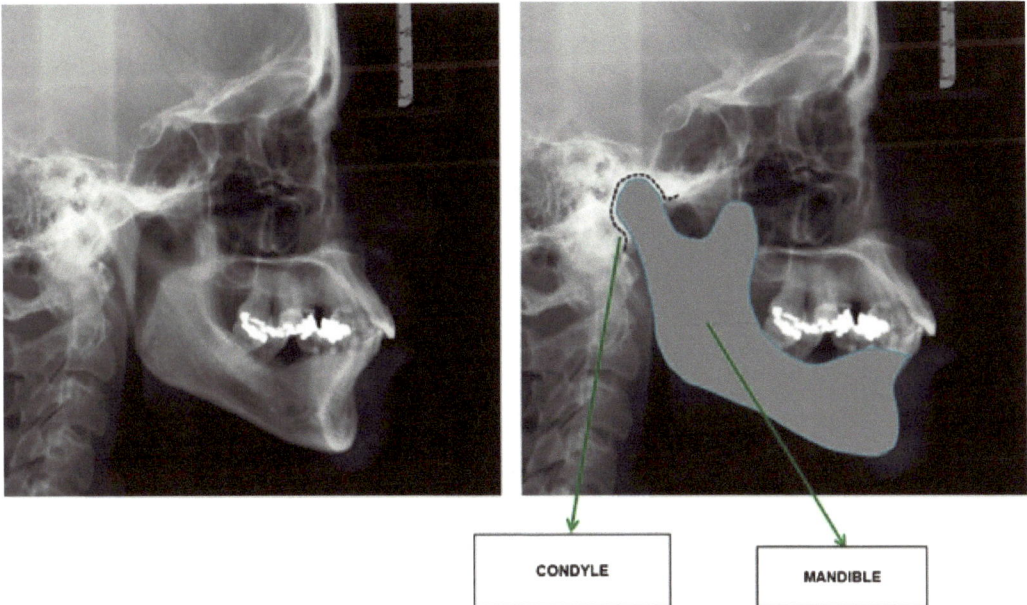

**Fig. (2).** Cephalometric Radiography.

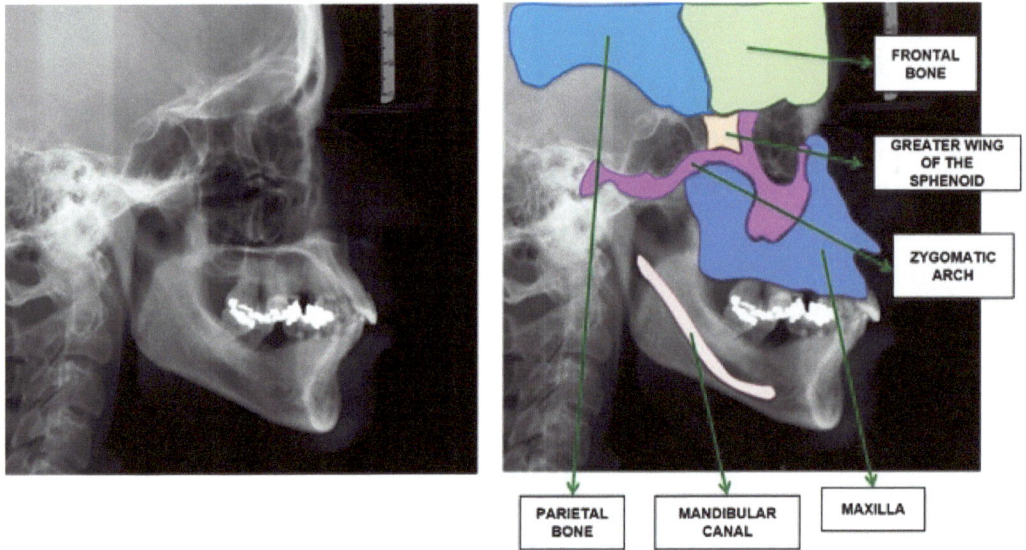

**Fig. (3).** Cephalometric Radiography.

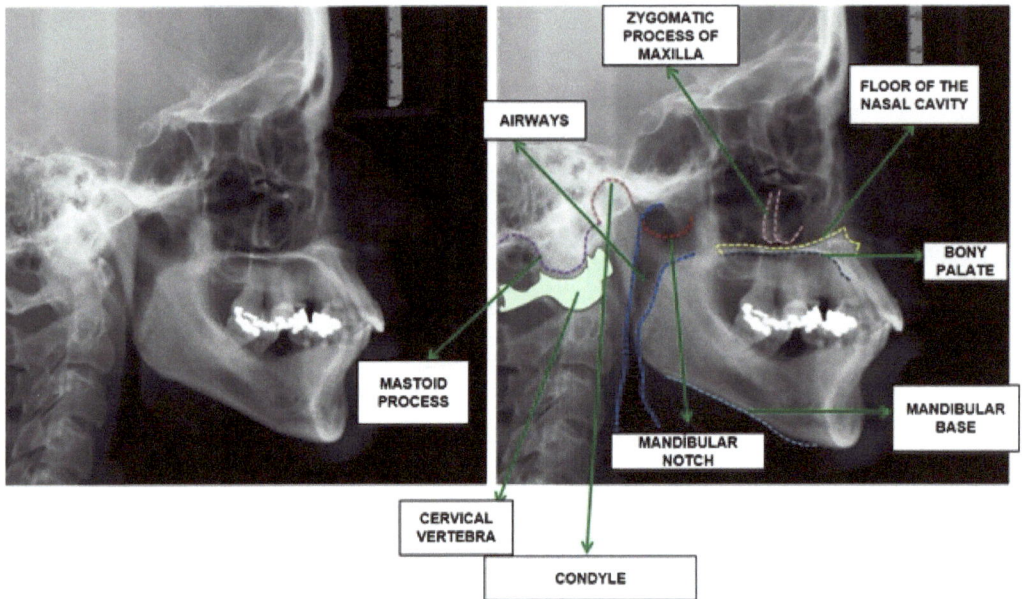

**Fig. (4).** Cephalometric Radiography.

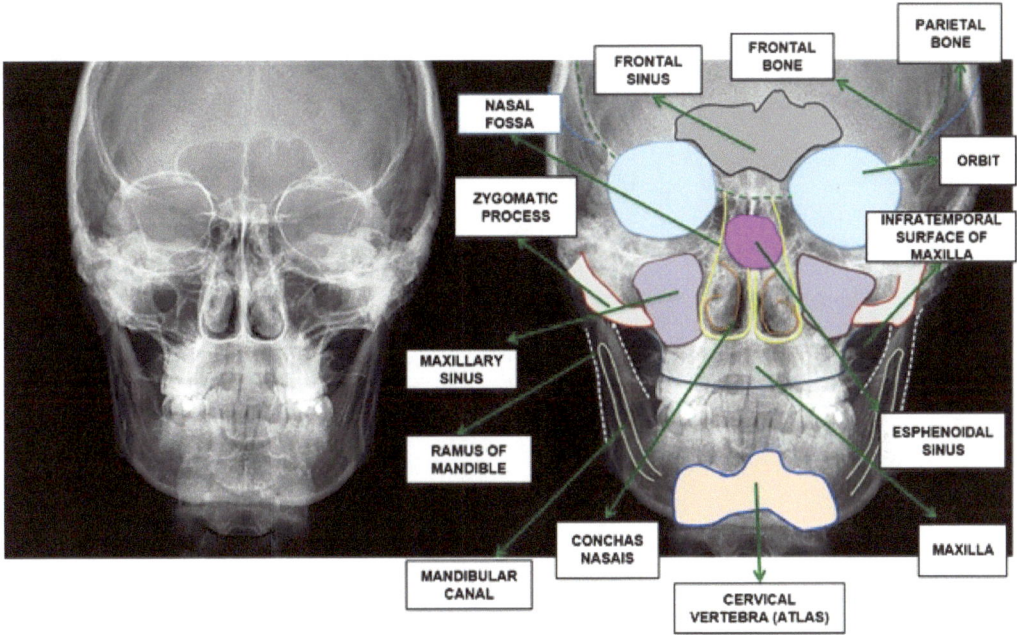

**Fig. (5).** Posterior Anterior (PA) Skull Radiograph (Caldwell).

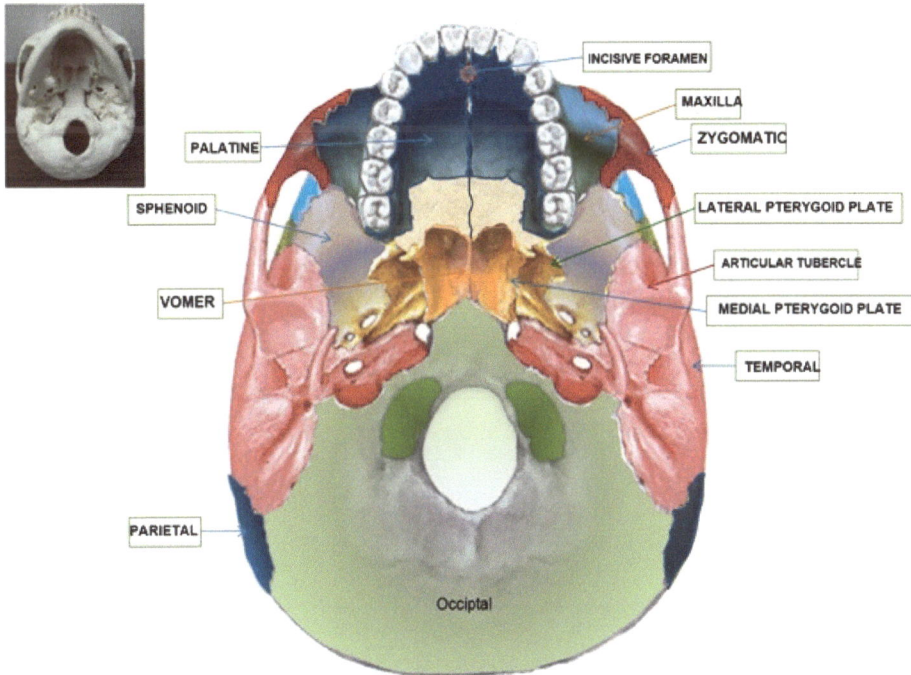

**Fig. (6).** Inferior View of Skull.

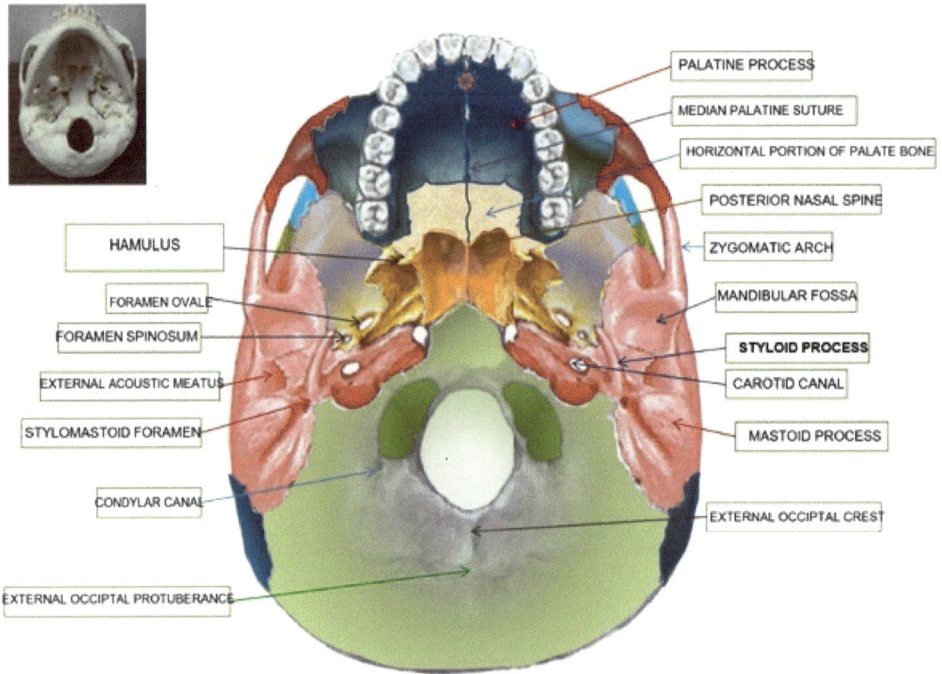

**Fig. (7).** Inferior View of Skull.

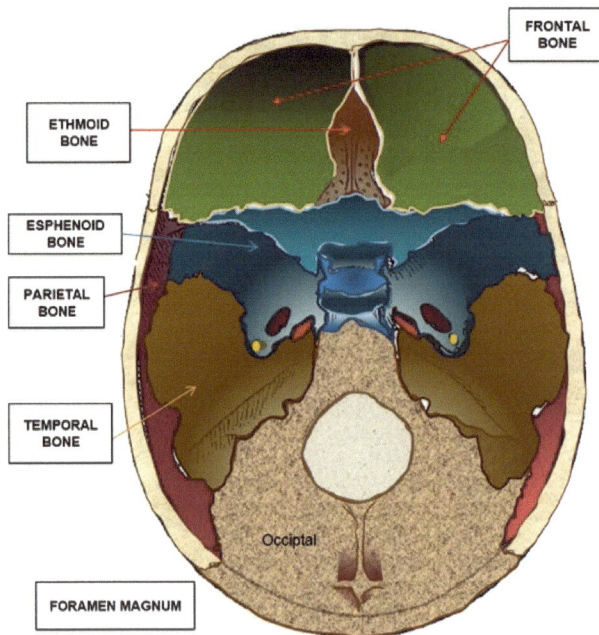

**Fig. (8).** Cross Section of Skull.

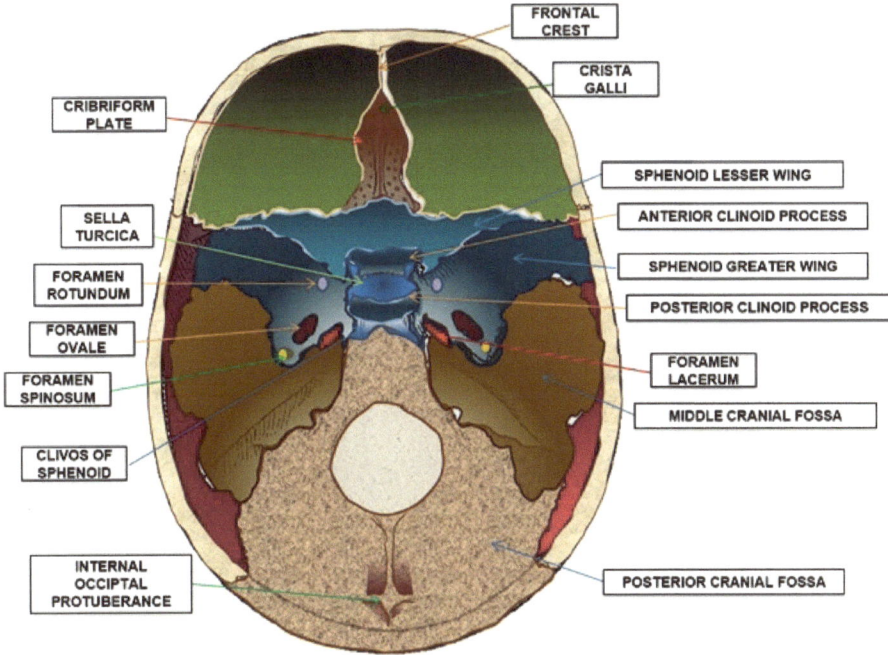

**Fig. (9).** Cross Section of Skull.

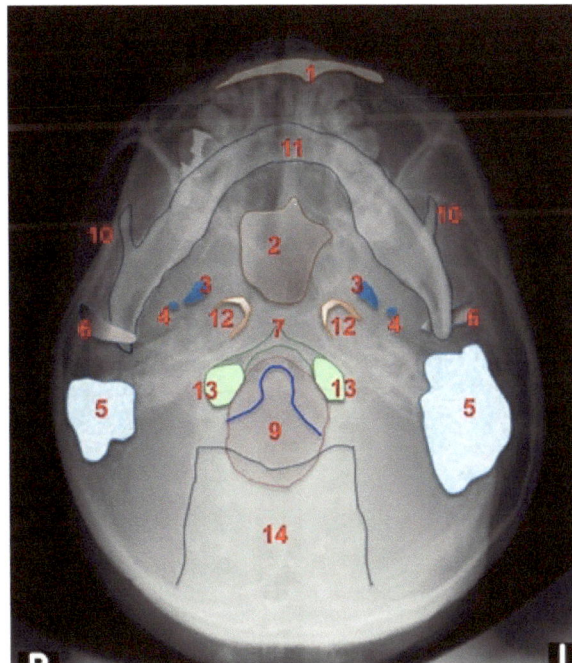

1 – FRONTAL SINUS

2 - ESPHENOIDAL SINUS

3 - OVAL FORAMEN

4 - FORAMEN SPINOSUM

5 - MASTOID CELLS

6 - CONDYLE

7 – ATLAS ANTERIOR ARCH

8 - DENS OF AXIS

9 - FORAMEN MAGNUM

10 - CORONOID APOPHYSIS

11 - MANDIBLE

12 - FORAMEN LACERUM

13 - OCCIPTAL CONDYLE

14 - SPINAL PROJECTION

**Fig. (10).** Hirtz Projection or Axial.

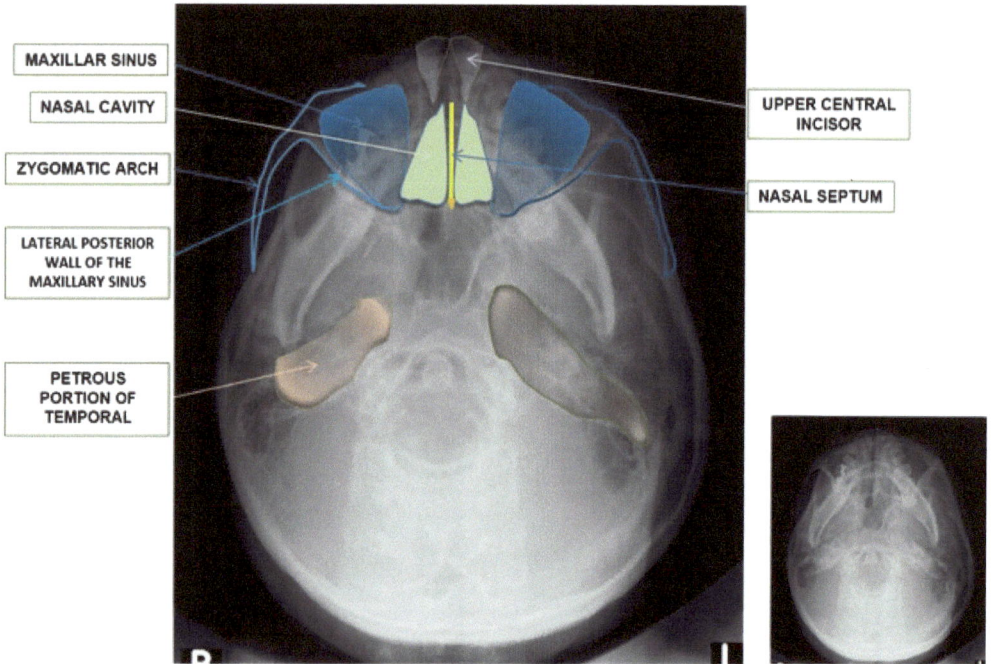

**Fig. (11).** Hirtz Projection or Axial.

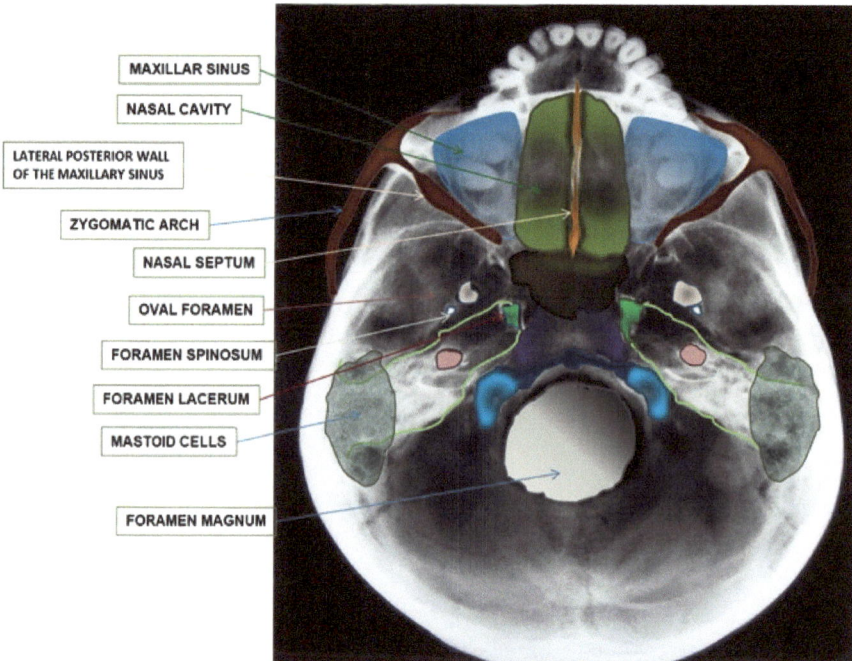

**Fig. (12).** Hirtz Projection or Axial.

The anterior fossa accommodates brain frontal lobe. The frontal bone forms the majority of the floor and in the middle region is crista galli and cribriform plate with numerous olfactory nerves as carriers for nasal cavity.

In the middle fossa is the Sella turcica. In greater wing of the sphenoid foramen ovale and foramen spinosum can be observed, which respectively pass mandibular nerve and the middle meningeal artery.

The foramen magnum is in the posterior fossa of the cranial base.

## PA projection – Waters [1 - 4]

The maxillary sinuses are best observed by Water's technique, inclusive of the inferior orbital base and can detect depression, erosions and small fractures. The oblique orbital lines represent anterior portions of the middle temporal fossa, the greater wing of the sphenoid bone. Maxillary sinus may have various shapes and sizes depending on the facial type, number of teeth and age. It has a tendency to invade the spaces left by missing teeth becoming developed in edentulous patients (Figs. **13-14**).

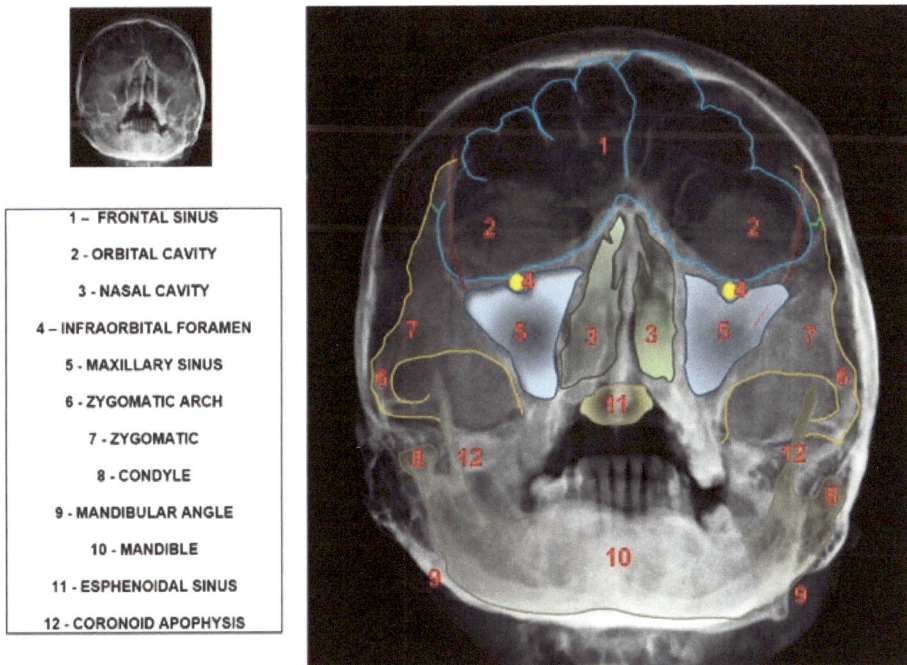

1 – FRONTAL SINUS

2 - ORBITAL CAVITY

3 - NASAL CAVITY

4 – INFRAORBITAL FORAMEN

5 - MAXILLARY SINUS

6 - ZYGOMATIC ARCH

7 - ZYGOMATIC

8 - CONDYLE

9 - MANDIBULAR ANGLE

10 - MANDIBLE

11 - ESPHENOIDAL SINUS

12 - CORONOID APOPHYSIS

**Fig. (13).** PA Waters.

1 – FRONTAL SINUS

2 - ORBITAL CAVITY

3 - NASAL CAVITY

4 - INFRATEMPORAL FOSSA

5 - MASTOID PROCESS

6 - MASTOID CELLS

7 - MANDIBULAR ANGLE

8 - CRISTA GALLI

9 - ETHMOIDAL SINUS

10 - NASAL SEPTUM

11 - ZIGOMATIC

12 - ESPHENOIDAL SINUS

13 - DENS OF AXIS

14 - CONDYLE

15 - CORONOID PROCESS

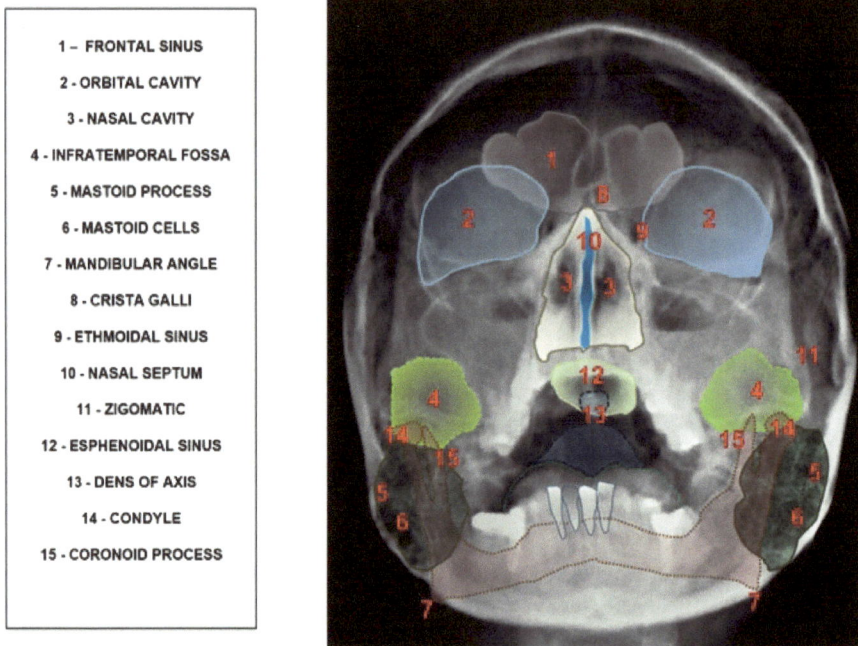

**Fig. (14).** PA Waters.

The sphenoid sinus can be seen in this projection with open mouth, can present with the morphology and varying sizes. Body and arch of the zygomatic bone can be clearly observed. Zygomatic-temporal suture appears as oblique radiolucent line that should not be confused as a fracture line.

Several conditions can cause thickening of the sinus mucosa to become visible radiographically. These are the allergic inflammation, chemical irritations, infections, *etc*.

The images show slight increase opacity around the sinus wall.

## Frontal View of Skull [1 - 4]

The most prominent facial bones subject to direct trauma are the zygomatic (sinking) and nasal (transverse). Fractures of the alveolar process in the anterior region are also common with shock or surgical trauma (Figs. **15-16**).

The maxillary sinus can present various shapes and sizes depending on the facial type, number of teeth and age. Tends to invade the spaces left by extracted teeth becoming developed in edentulous patients (Figs. **18-20**).

## Panoramic Radiograph [1 - 4]

Panoramic radiograph – PR (also called ortopantomography) is a technique for producing a single image of the facial structures that includes both maxillary and the mandibular dental arches and their supporting structures (Figs. **21-27**).

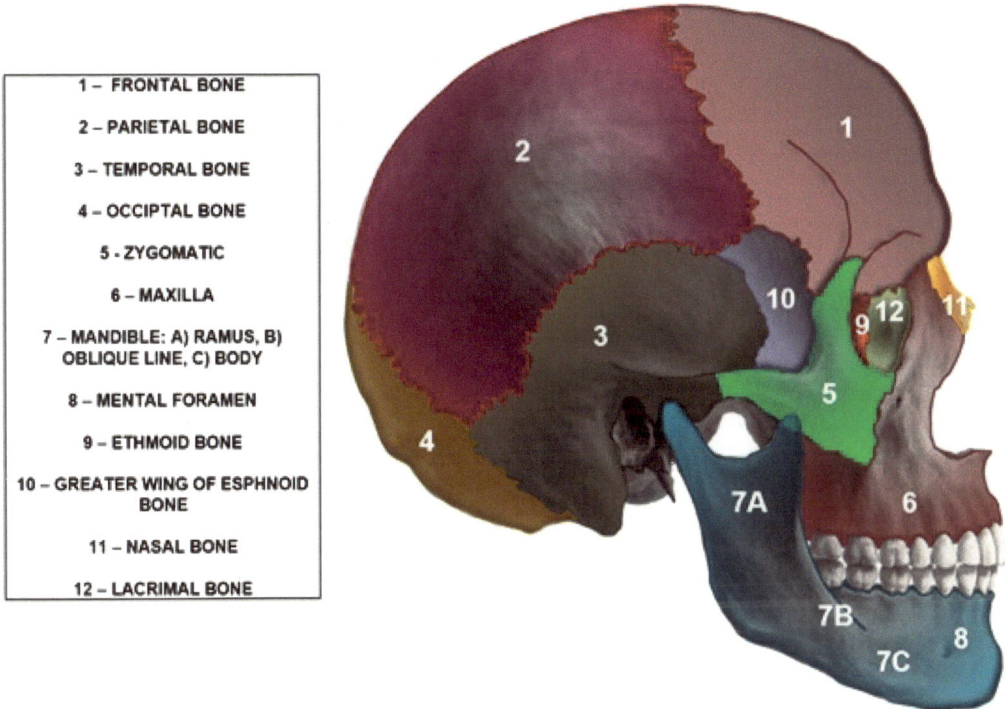

| 1 – FRONTAL BONE |
| --- |
| 2 – PARIETAL BONE |
| 3 – TEMPORAL BONE |
| 4 – OCCIPTAL BONE |
| 5 - ZYGOMATIC |
| 6 – MAXILLA |
| 7 – MANDIBLE: A) RAMUS, B) OBLIQUE LINE, C) BODY |
| 8 – MENTAL FORAMEN |
| 9 – ETHMOID BONE |
| 10 – GREATER WING OF ESPHNOID BONE |
| 11 – NASAL BONE |
| 12 – LACRIMAL BONE |

**Fig. (15).** Lateral View of Skull.

Temporalmandibular Joint (TMJ) is a bilateral and synovial joint consists of bony parts: the condyle, articular tubercle and glenoid fossa (Figs. **17, 28-35**).

In this technique, the patient remains motionless while the x-ray source and the radiographic sensors move in opposite direction at one or more centers of rotation. These pivot points can be internal or external focal area. Focal area tomography or "focal plane" or "image layer" or "cutting plan" is the plan that is not blurred in the radiographic image. PR is produced using tomographic curved surface and is performed by rotating a narrow radiation beam in a horizontal plane around a point / virtual axis (called rotation center) positioned within the oral cavity. Film / sensor head and move in the opposite direction around the patient, which remains stationary.

| |
|---|
| 1 – FRONTAL BONE |
| 2 - GLABELA |
| 3 – PARIETAL BONE |
| 4 - NASAL BONE |
| 5 – VOMER |
| 6 - ESPHENOID |
| 7 – SUPERIOR ORBITAL FISSURE |
| 8 – PERPENDICULAR PLATE OF ETHMOID |
| 9 - MAXILLA |
| 10 – ZIGOMATIC BONE |
| 11 – TEMPORAL BONE |
| 12 - MANDIBLE |
| 13 - MANDIBULAR ANGLE |
| 14 - MENTAL FORAMEN |
| 15 - MASTOID PROCESS |

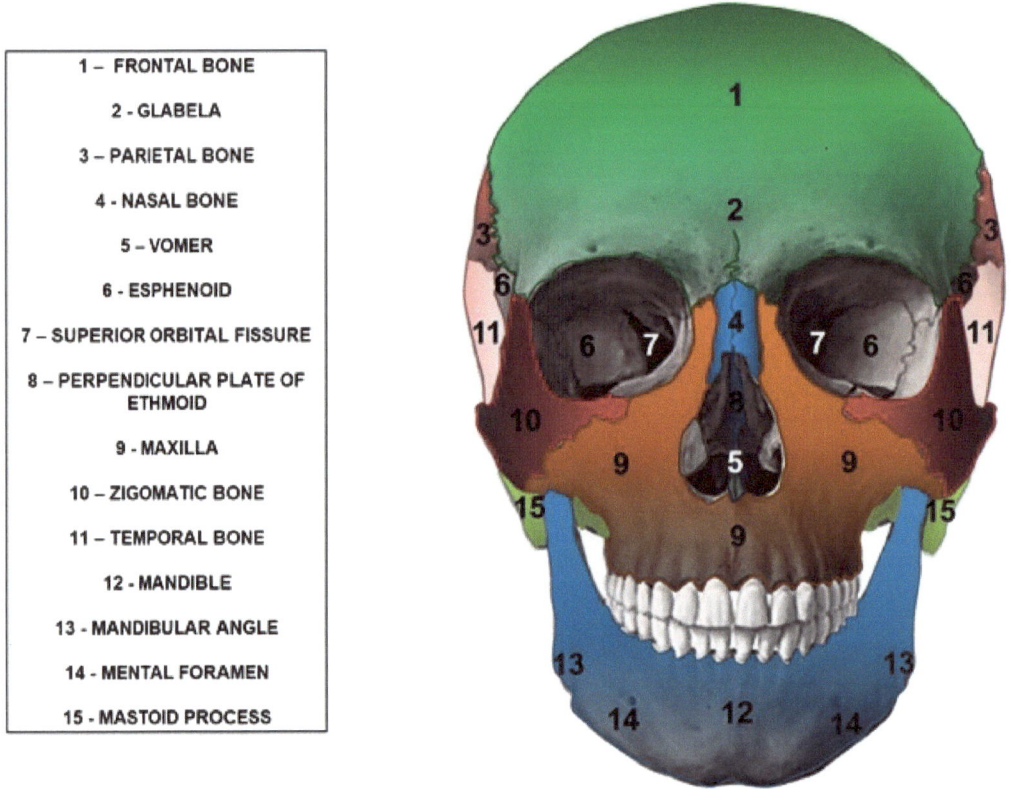

**Fig. (16).** Frontal View of Skull.

PR is an important diagnostic test widely used in dentistry as well as intra-oral examinations. Thus, allowing the observation of large areas (maxillomandibular) in case of normal or pathological conditions, possibility of x-ray in cases of severe nausea and trismus, narrow or shallow arch mouth floor. It also has the added benefit of reducing the radiation dose compared with intra-oral radiographs of the entire mouth.

PR is different from intraoral images and require a different approach. Recognizing normal anatomical structures in PR is a challenge due to complex medium third of face anatomy and several anatomical structures superposition. Artifacts appear in image most often due to patient motion at the time of examination, wrong patient position and unusual patient anatomy. The absence of any anatomical structure can be the most important finding of the exam.

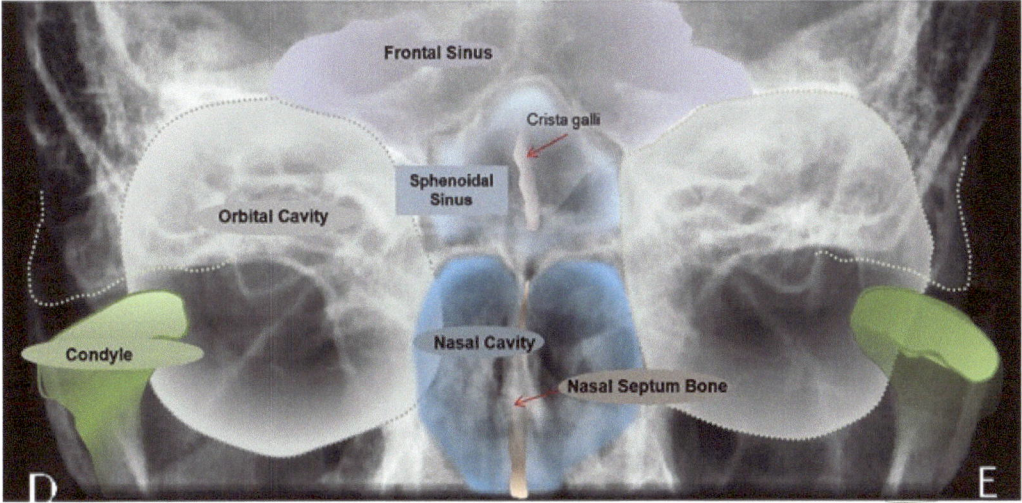

**Fig. (17).** Temporalmandibular Joint (TMJ).

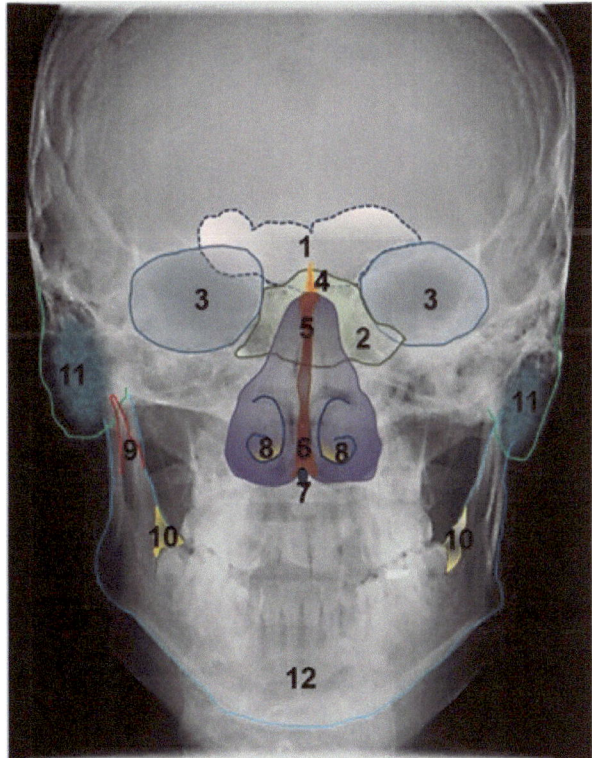

1 – FRONTAL SINUS

2 – ESPHENOIDAL SINUS

3 - ORBITAL CAVITY

4 - CRISTA GALLI

5 - PERPENDICULAR PLATE OF ETHMOID

6 – VOMER

7 – ANTERIOR NASAL SPINE

8 - INFERIOR NASAL CONCHA

9 - CORONOID PROCESS

10 - RETROMOLAR TRIGONE

11 - MASTOID PROCESS

12 - MANDIBLE

**Fig. (18).** PA.

1 – FRONTAL SINUS
2 - CRISTA GALLI
3 - ETHMOIDAL SINUS
4 - ORBITAL CAVITY
5 – FRONTOZYGOMATIC SUTURE
6 - NASAL SEPTUM
7 - INFERIOR NASAL CONCHA
8 - DENS OF AXIS
9 - ATLANTOAXIAL JOINT
10 - CONDYLE
11 - CORONOID PROCESS
12 - RETROMOLAR TRIGONE

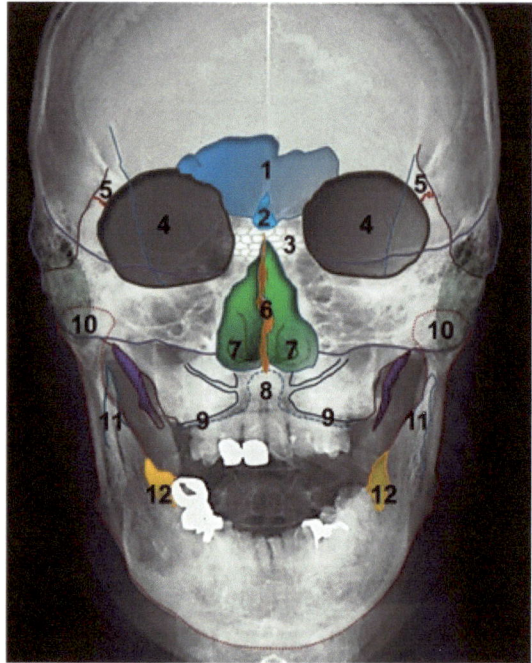

**Fig. (19).** PA.

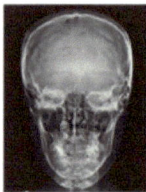

1 – ESPHENOIDAL SINUS
2 - ORBITAL CAVITY
3 – MASTOID PROCESS
4 - NASAL SEPTUM
5 – MAXILLARY SINUS

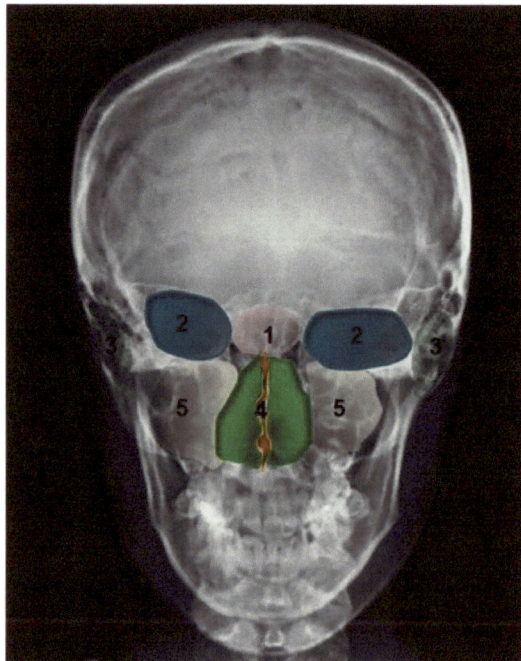

**Fig. (20).** PA.

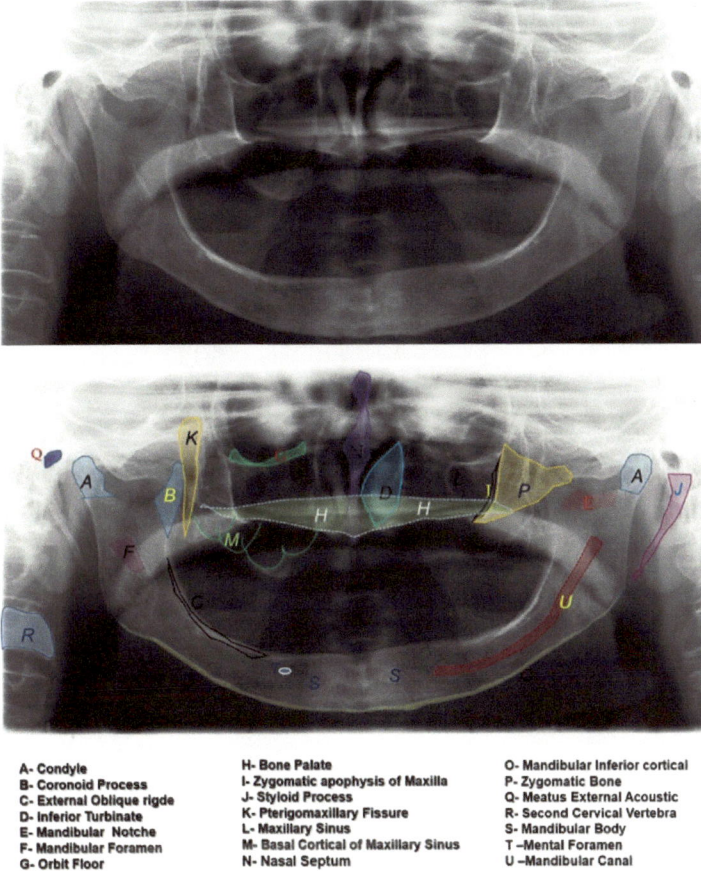

A- Condyle
B- Coronoid Process
C- External Oblique rigde
D- Inferior Turbinate
E- Mandibular Notche
F- Mandibular Foramen
G- Orbit Floor

H- Bone Palate
I- Zygomatic apophysis of Maxilla
J- Styloid Process
K- Pterigomaxillary Fissure
L- Maxillary Sinus
M- Basal Cortical of Maxillary Sinus
N- Nasal Septum

O- Mandibular Inferior cortical
P- Zygomatic Bone
Q- Meatus External Acoustic
R- Second Cervical Vertebra
S- Mandibular Body
T –Mental Foramen
U –Mandibular Canal

**Fig. (21).** Panoramic Radiograph.

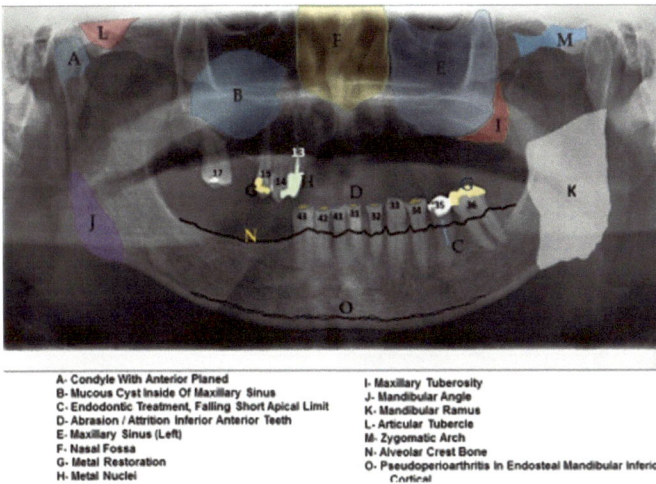

A- Condyle With Anterior Planed
B- Mucous Cyst Inside Of Maxillary Sinus
C- Endodontic Treatment, Falling Short Apical Limit
D- Abrasion / Attrition Inferior Anterior Teeth
E- Maxillary Sinus (Left)
F- Nasal Fossa
G- Metal Restoration
H- Metal Nuclei

I- Maxillary Tuberosity
J- Mandibular Angle
K- Mandibular Ramus
L- Articular Tubercle
M- Zygomatic Arch
N- Alveolar Crest Bone
O- Pseudoperioarthritis In Endosteal Mandibular Inferior
   Cortical

**Fig. (22).** Panoramic Radiograph.

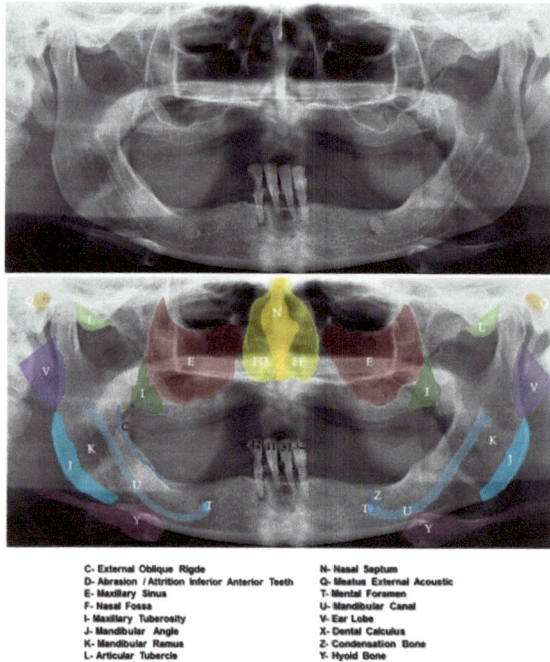

C- External Oblique Rigde
D- Abrasion / Attrition Inferior Anterior Teeth
E- Maxillary Sinus
F- Nasal Fossa
I- Maxillary Tuberosity
J- Mandibular Angle
K- Mandibular Ramus
L- Articular Tubercle

N- Nasal Septum
Q- Meatus External Acoustic
T- Mental Foramen
U- Mandibular Canal
V- Ear Lobe
X- Dental Calculus
Z- Condensation Bone
Y- Hyoid Bone

**Fig. (23).** Panoramic Radiograph.

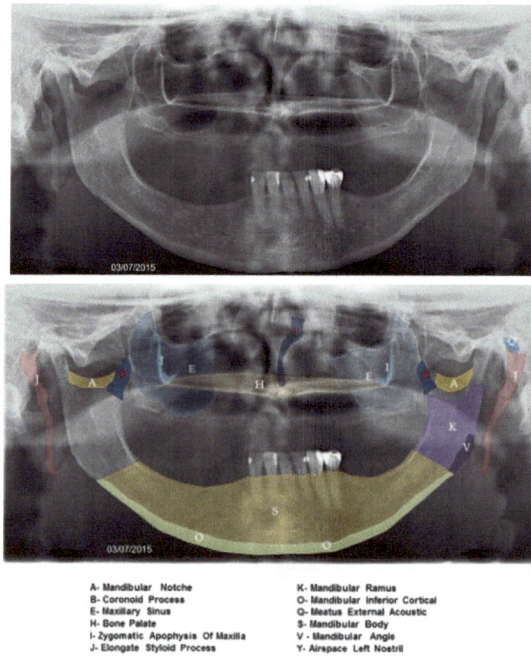

A- Mandibular Notche
B- Coronoid Process
E- Maxillary Sinus
H- Bone Palate
I- Zygomatic Apophysis Of Maxilla
J- Elongate Styloid Process

K- Mandibular Ramus
O- Mandibular Inferior Cortical
Q- Meatus External Acoustic
S- Mandibular Body
V - Mandibular Angle
Y- Airspace Left Nostril

**Fig. (24).** Panoramic Radiograph.

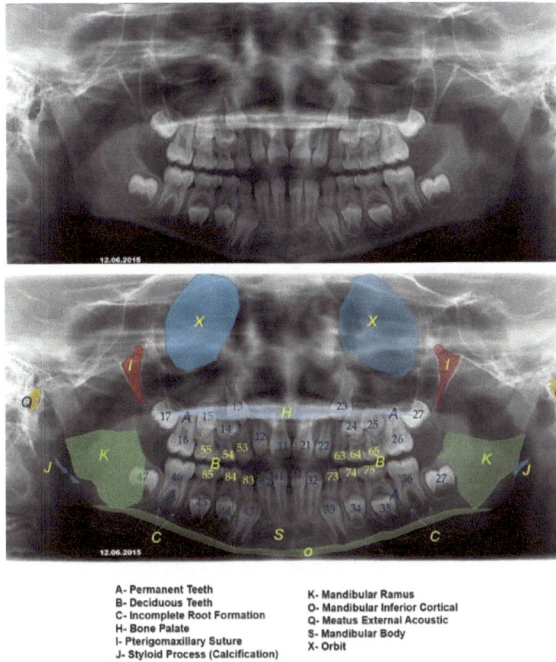

A- Permanent Teeth
B- Deciduous Teeth
C- Incomplete Root Formation
H- Bone Palate
I- Pterigomaxilary Suture
J- Styloid Process (Calcification)

K- Mandibular Ramus
O- Mandibular Inferior Cortical
Q- Meatus External Acoustic
S- Mandibular Body
X- Orbit

**Fig. (25).** Panoramic Radiograph.

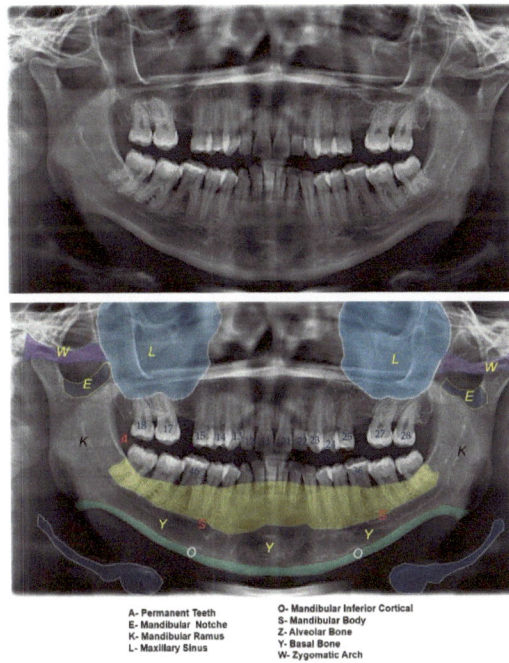

A- Permanent Teeth
E- Mandibular Notche
K- Mandibular Ramus
L- Maxillary Sinus

O- Mandibular Inferior Cortical
S- Mandibular Body
Z- Alveolar Bone
Y- Basal Bone
W- Zygomatic Arch

**Fig. (26).** Panoramic Radiograph.

A- Permanent Teeth
AA- Middle Cranial Fossa
BB- Submandibular Fovea
K- Mandibular Ramus
CC- Plastic Restoration
DD- Alveolar Bone Crest

EE- Dental Follicle, Containing Germ Tooth 3ªm
FF- Nasal Airspace Nostrils.
GG- Infraorbital Foramen
L- Maxillary Sinus
O- Mandibular Inferior Cortical
V- Ear Lobe
X- Orbit

**Fig. (27).** Panoramic Radiograph.

**Fig. (28).** Temporomandibular Joint Radiograph – Right side with mouth closed.

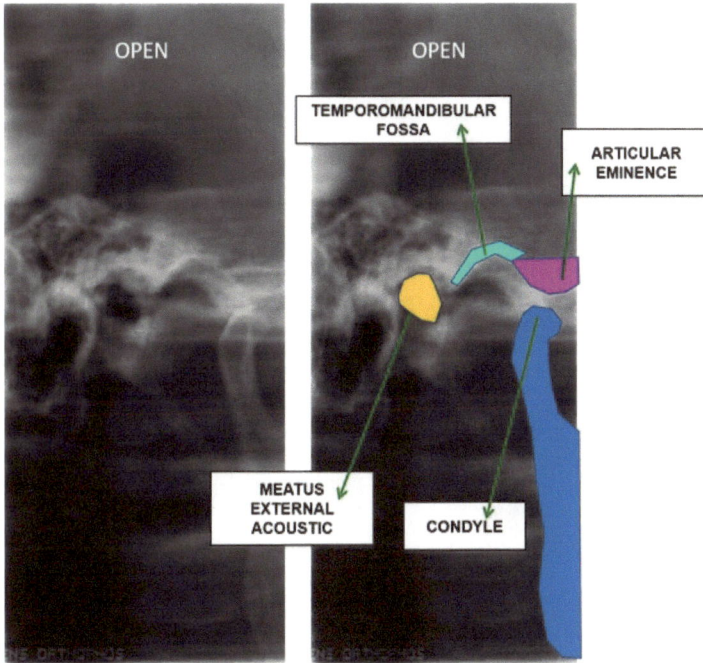

**Fig. (29).** Temporomandibular Joint Radiograph – Right side with mouth open.

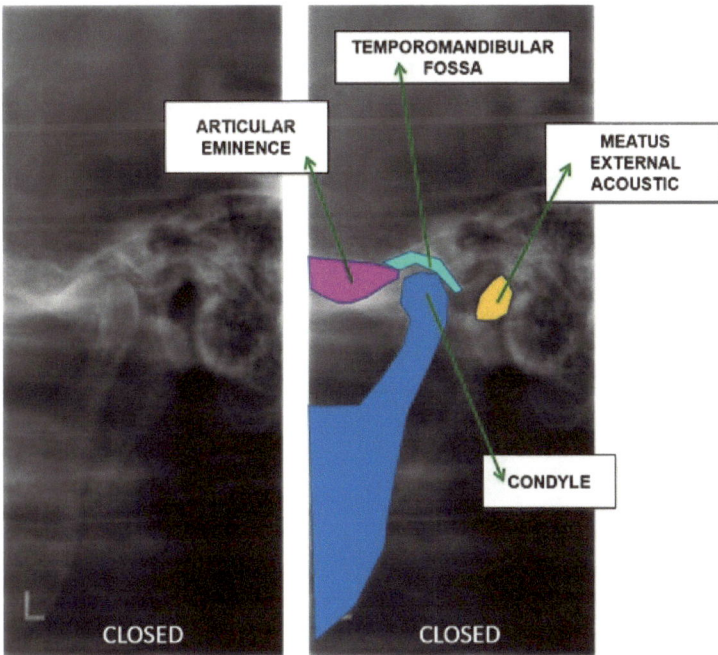

**Fig. (30).** Temporomandibular Joint Radiograph – Left side with mouth closed.

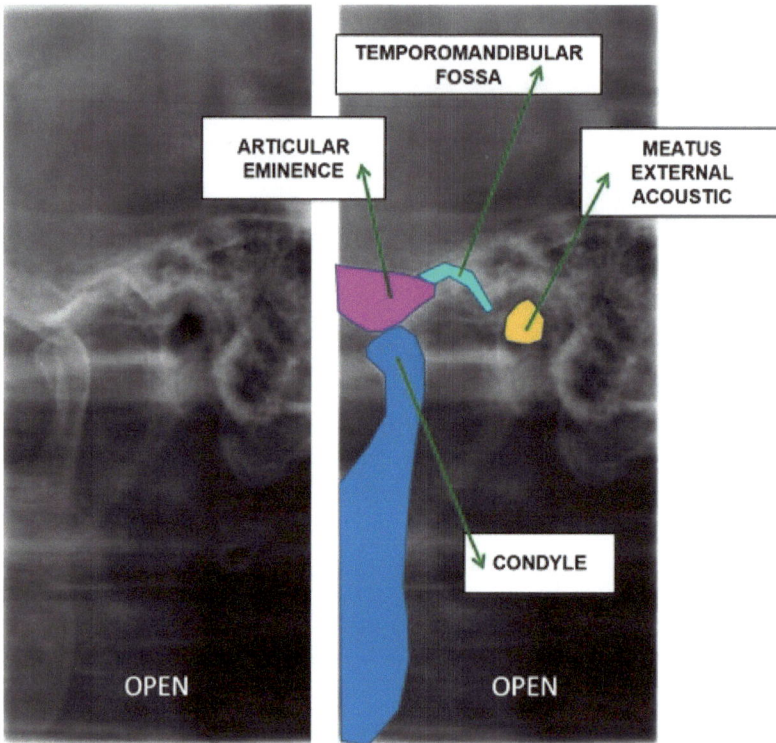

**Fig. (31).** Temporomandibular Joint Radiograph – Left side with mouth open.

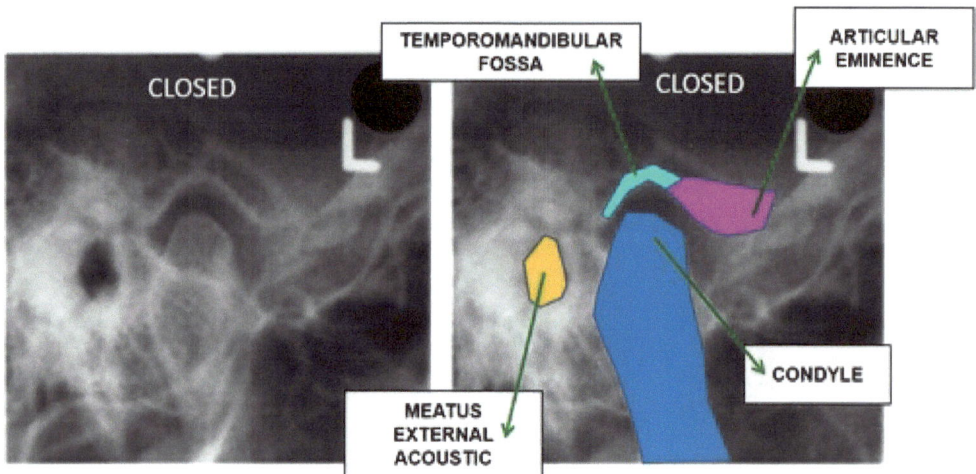

**Fig. (32).** Temporomandibular Joint Radiograph – Left side with mouth closed.

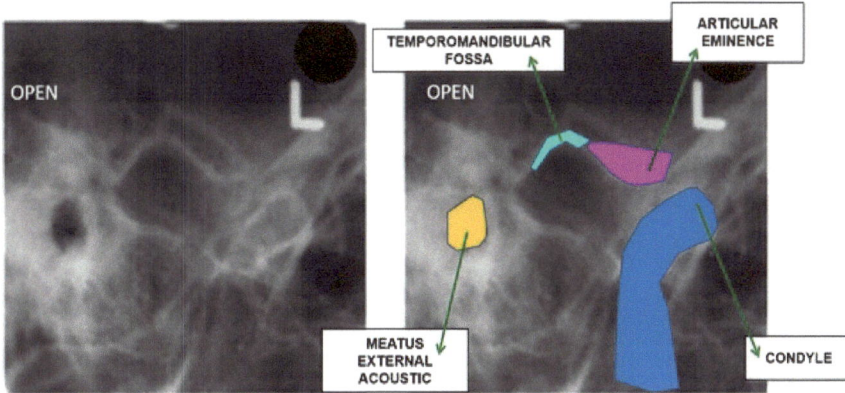

**Fig. (33).** Temporomandibular Joint Radiograph – Left side with mouth open.

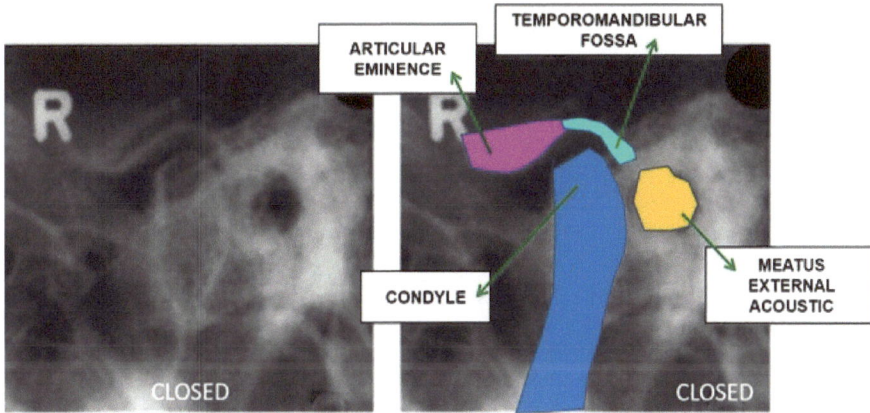

**Fig. (34).** Temporomandibular Joint Radiograph – Right side with mouth closed.

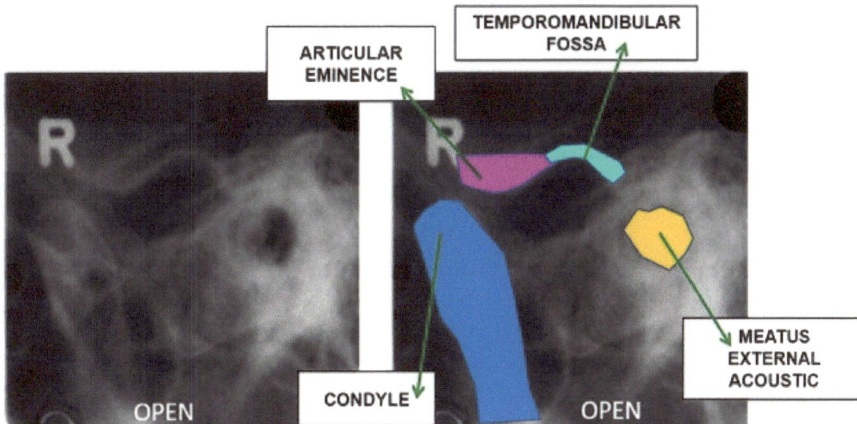

**Fig. (35).** Temporomandibular Joint Radiograph – Right side with mouth open.

## CONSENT FOR PUBLICATION

Not applicable.

## CONFLICT OF INTEREST

The author declares no conflict of interest, financial or otherwise.

## ACKNOWLEDGEMENTS

Decleared none.

## REFERENCES

[1]   Freitas A, Rosa JE, Souza IF. Odontologic Radiographic. 6th ed., São Paulo: Artes Médicas 2004.

[2]   Madeira MC. Face Anatomy. 7th ed., São Paulo: Sarvier 2010.

[3]   Watanabe PC, Arita ES. Radiologia Odontológica e Imaginologia. 1st ed., Rio de Janeiro: Elsevier 2012.

[4]   White SC, Pharoah MJ. Oral Radiology – Principles and Interpretation. 7th ed., Rio de Janeiro: Elsevier 2015.

# CHAPTER 5

# Pathologies and Anatomical Abnormalities

Plauto C. A. Watanabe*, Emiko S. Arita, Angela J. Camargo and Marina G. Baladi

*School of Dentistry of Ribeirão Preto, University of São Paulo, São Paulo, Brazil*

**Abstract:** Abstract: In order to evaluate the pathological condition, the radiographic image of the normal anatomical structure must be correctly known. The evaluation of pathological lesions of the head and neck regions involves routine use of radiographs in the main attempt to determine the nature of the abnormality and / or the pathological process. In the dental clinic in Brazil, in general, the dental surgeon mainly performs the intraoral radiographic examinations, since he works in his routine of attendance with intraoral X-ray equipment. Thus, it has been the protocol of service to request a panoramic radiography, when the patient first consulted, based on the clinical examination and the request for care. This is very important so that the professional can arrive at a differential diagnosis as close as possible. The reality is that we will not always have the pathognomonic signs of the pathologies (main characteristics of the lesion).

**Keywords:** Dental anomalies, Maxillo-mandibular complex, Panoramic radiography.

A variety of dental abnormalities are associated with defects in the development of teeth caused by factors such as heredity, local, systemic or traumatic. These disturbances in the anatomical structures, result in a deviation from the normal, denominating these alterations of anomalies. Numerous systems have been used to classify dental anomalies as size, number, structure.

## QUANTITATIVE CHANGES (NUMBER) [1]

Supernumerary teeth is the increase of the number of teeth in the dental arch. In general, teeth are smaller than the teeth of the region where they appear and may have anatomical variation (Figs. **1-3**).

Agenesis is the absence of the formation of the dental germ and can occur in deciduous and permanent dentition (Fig. **4**).

---

* **Corresponding author Plauto C. A. Watanabe:** School of Dentistry of Ribeirão Preto, University of São Paulo, São Paulo, Brazil; Tel: 55-16-33153993; E-mail: watanabe@forp.usp.br

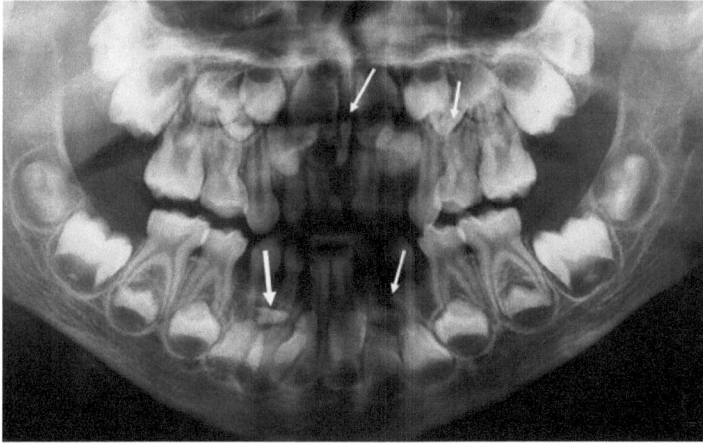

**Fig. (1).** Supernumerary teeth signaled with arrows.

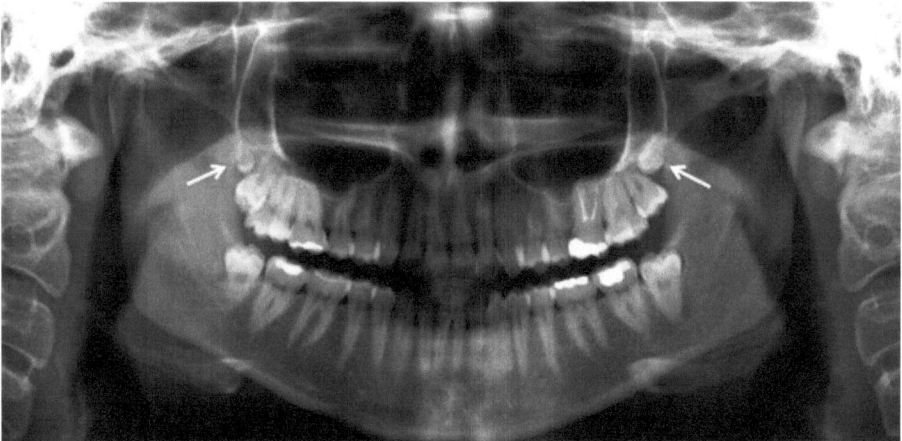

**Fig. (2).** Supernumerary teeth signaled with arrows.

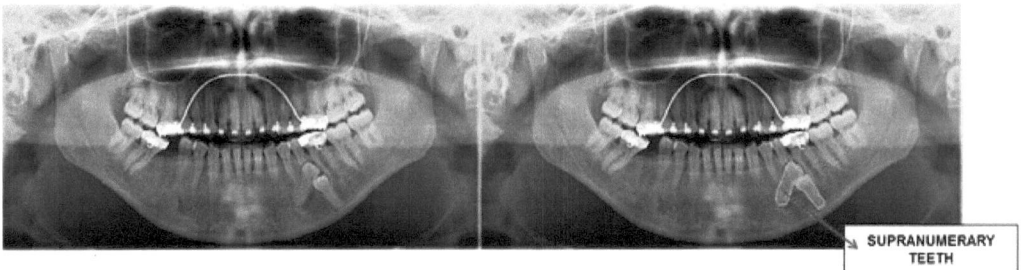

**Fig. (3).** Supernumerary teeth.

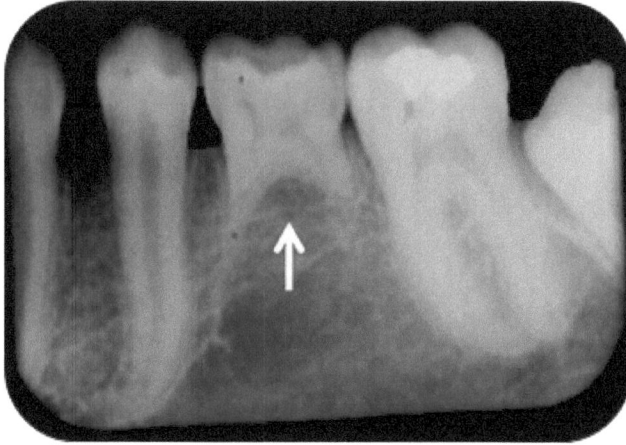

**Fig. (4).** Agenesis of premolar signaled with arrows.

## SIZE ANOMALIES [1]

Microdontia is an anomaly that compromises the volume of the tooth, being able to be of three varieties: *genuine generalized microdontia*, a rare condition that encompasses all dentitions, where all teeth are well formed but smaller; *relative generalized microdontia*, the jaws are very large, they simulate a decrease in the size of the teeth, when, in fact, they are normal; and *unidental microdontia* is a fairly common condition where only one tooth is involved (Fig. **5**).

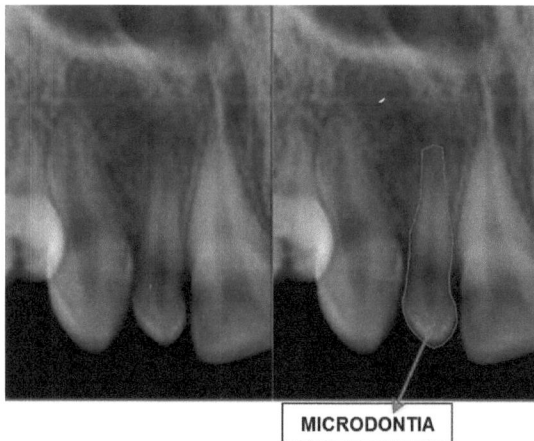

MICRODONTIA

**Fig. (5).** Microdontia of lateral.

Macrodontia, is the opposite of microdontia, obeying the same classification, with the variant that true generalized macrodontia is associated with pituitary gigantism, and isolated macrodontia affecting only one tooth. "Conoid tooth" represents a form of microdontia that can be uni or multi dental. The tooth loses its normal morphological characteristics to acquire a conical shape, which can cover only the crown, as well as the root.

## MORPHOLOGICAL CHANGES (SHAPE) [1]

Form anomalies originate during the morphodifferentiation stage and are manifested as alternations in the shape of the crown and root. Hereditary patterns include autosomal dominant inheritance and polygenic.

Gemination results of a developmental aberration of ectoderm and the mesoderm, the teeth germ divides and results a "two teeth", with two crowns or one large partially separated crown, can be share a pulp chamber and root canal, affected most the permanent maxillary incisors (Figs. **6**, **7**).

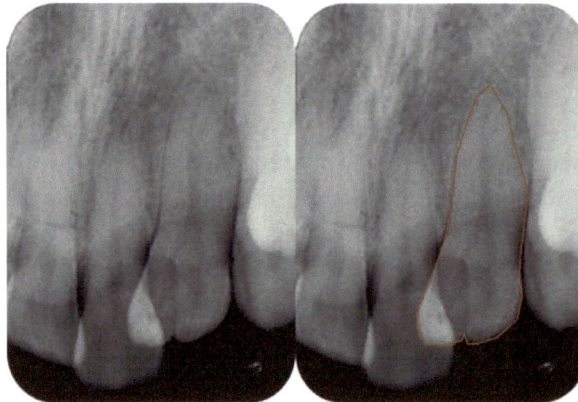

**Fig. (6).** Gemination tooth.

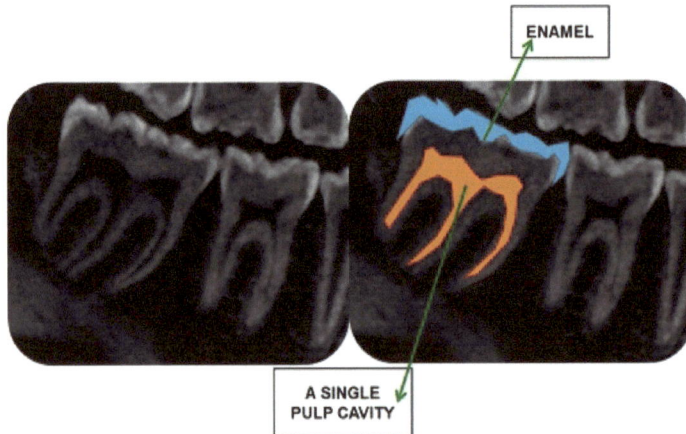

**Fig. (7).** A rare case for discussion: fusion or gemination?

Fusion is a union of two teeth as a result of some physical force or pressure, can be present with only one pulp chamber and a confluence of enamel and dentine as in gemination, or there may be two separate pulp chambers and union only of the dentine, involving permanent dentition are very rare 0–0.8%, with the majority of cases seen in anterior teeth, the congenital absence of the adjacent tooth from the dental arch can be differentiated fusion from germination (Figs. **6-8**).

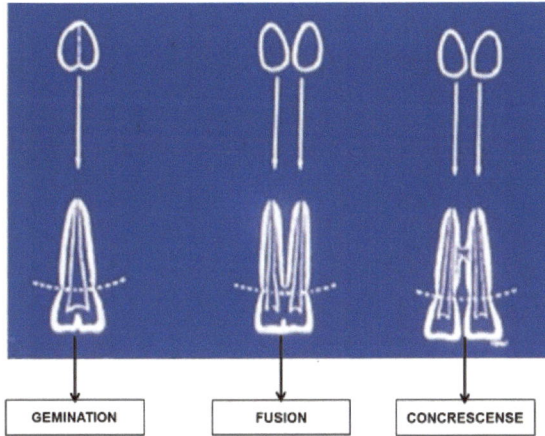

**Fig. (8).** Classification of morphological changes.

Concrescence are teeth that are adhered by cement, without the involvement of dentin. It is not possible to differentiate in the radiographic image.

Dilaceration refers to an abnormal curvature of the root during its development and may be the result of an episode of trauma in the deciduous dentition (Figs. **9**, **10**).

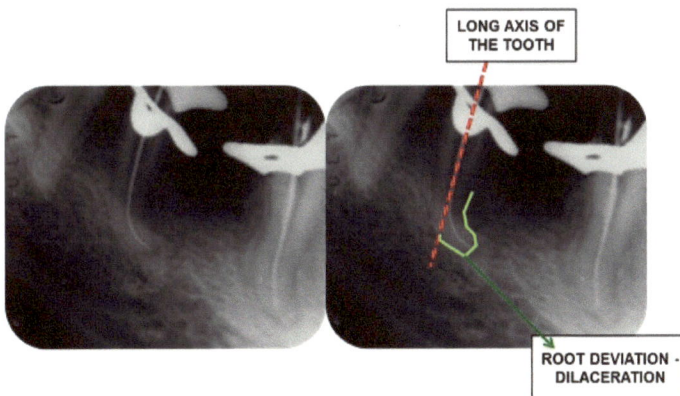

**Fig. (9).** Dilaceration Premolar root.

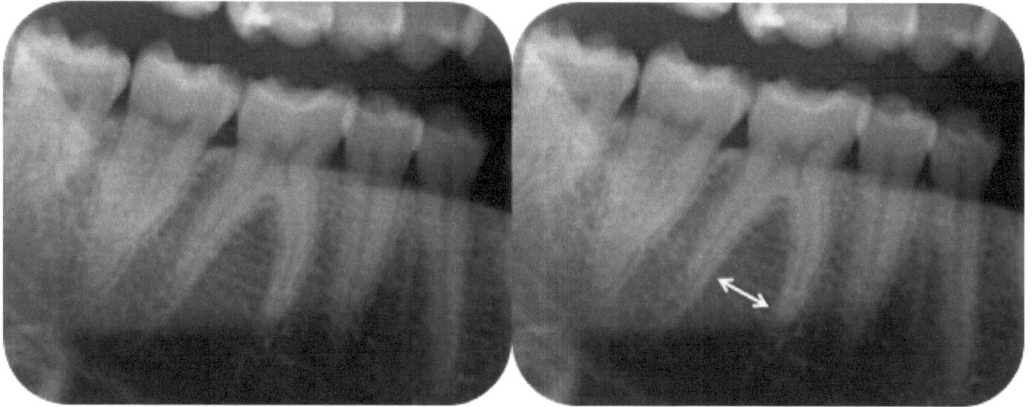

**Fig. (10).** Divergence Molar root (1rsMolar) and dilaceration (2ndMolar).

Dens Invaginatus is a variation in dental development, possibly due to invagination of the dental coronary surface, prior to calcification, interruption of lingual fossa development, or a proliferation of enamel organ cells within the dental papilla (Fig. **11**).

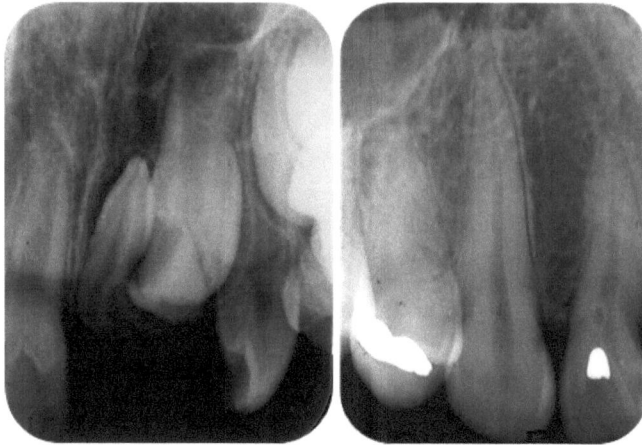

**Fig. (11).** Two different cases of Dens Invaginatus.

Evagination is an extra cusp, usually in the central fossil or groove of a posterior tooth, or in the cingulate region of a central or lateral incisor. In the incisors, these evaginations appear in conoid form, and can reach the level of the incisal edge.

Taurodontism is a hereditary disorder, in which the pulp chamber presents extraordinarily great, being able to extend to the area that would be of the roots (Fig. **12**).

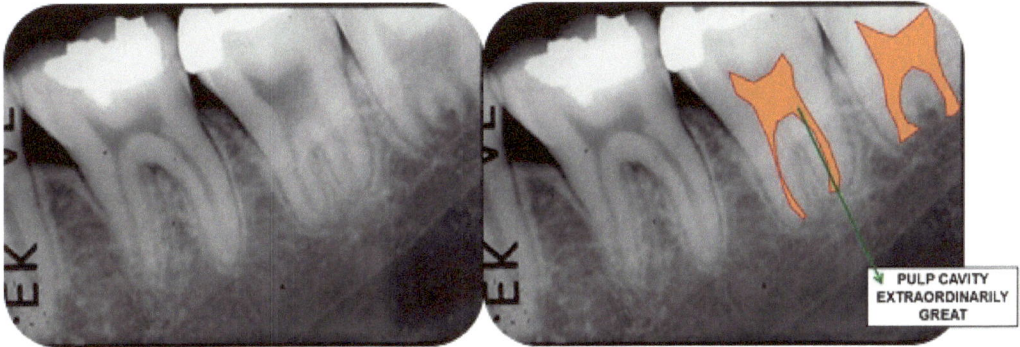

PULP CAVITY
EXTRAORDINARILY
GREAT

**Fig. (12).** Taurodontism.

Supernumerary roots are accessories and deviate from the normal pattern of specific teeth (Figs. **13**, **14**).

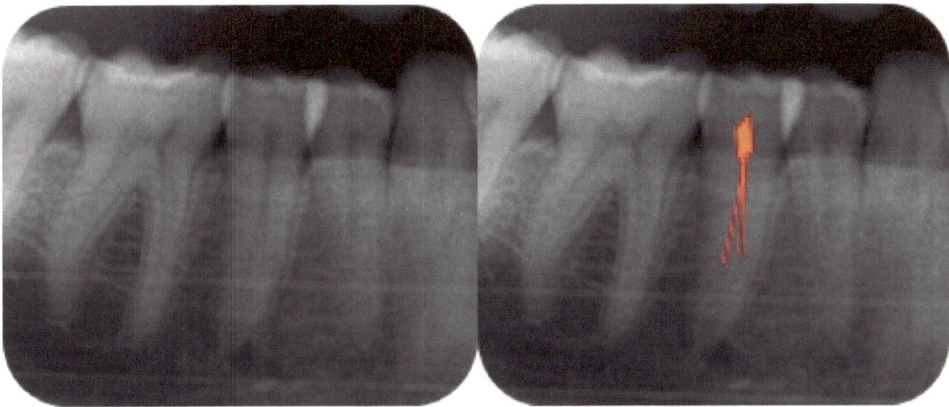

**Fig. (13).** Supernumerary roots.

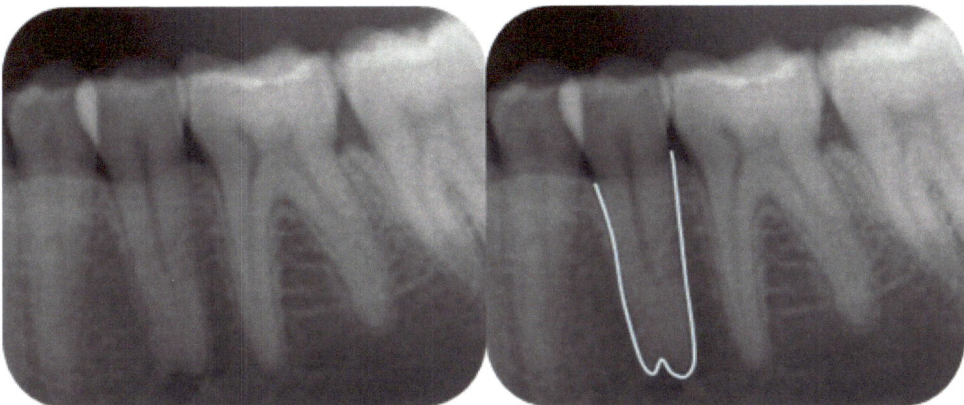

**Fig. (14).** Supernumerary roots.

## ANOMALIES OF STRUCTURE [1]

Enamel hypoplasia is defective or partial formation of the enamel structure of the teeth being able to vary from white spots, generalized stain, loss of structure forming cavities or grooves.

Turner's tooth is an enamel hypoplasia of the permanent teeth caused by trauma or local infection of the deciduous tooth.

Hutchinson's Tooth is a hypoplasia caused by congenital syphilis reaching the incisors and molars which are called mulberry molar.

Imperfect amelogenesis is a genetic anomaly that the enamel structure of deciduous and permanent teeth is hypoplastic. Radiographically depending on the degree of severity the enamel may be absent or with a thin layer (Fig. **15**).

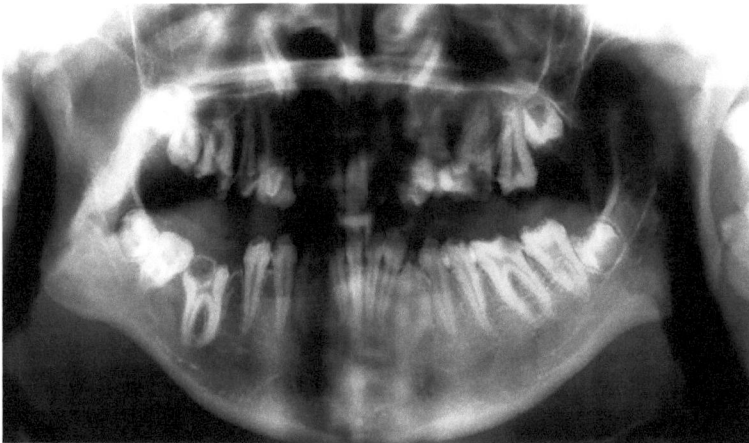

**Fig. (15).** Imperfect amelogenesis.

Imperfect dentinogenesis is a hereditary characteristic that affects the development of dentinal tissue, often accompanied by similar changes in the bones. Radiographically the appearance is typical: obliteration, by calcified tissues, total or partial of the chambers and pulp ducts, resulting from the continuous formation of dentin, and presenting short and conical roots.

## CONCLUSION

The preciousness in the study and knowledge of the anatomical structures, provides security for the discernment of possible pathologies and abnormalities. In clinical practice professionals who have good knowledge of anatomy and its borders feels safe to discern between the healthy and diseased, even if do not know the definitive diagnosis, know to search for plausible solutions.

## CONSENT FOR PUBLICATION

Not applicable.

## CONFLICT OF INTEREST

Radiographic material of the NACEDO - Nucleus of Support to Culture and Extension in Dental Diagnosis of the Pro-Rectory of Culture and University Extension (PRCExU / USP). Crowded at the School of Dentistry of Ribeirão Preto / University of São Paulo.

## ACKNOWLEDGEMENTS

NACEDO-PRCExU/USP

## REFERENCE

[1]     Watanabe PC, Arita ES. Odontologic Imaginology and Radiology. 1st ed., Rio de Janeiro: Elsevier 2012.

# SUBJECT INDEX

## A

Abnormalities, dental 77
Agenesis 77, 79
Alveolar bone 21, 22, 27, 41, 44, 45, 46
Alveolar bone crest 7, 21
Alveolar crest 44, 46, 47
  cortical 46
Alveolar crest fibers 44
Anatomical Abnormalities 7, 77, 79, 81, 83,
    85
Anatomical accidents 56
Anatomical accuracy 2
Anatomical feature, unique 49
Anatomical repair 53
Anatomical structures 1, 3, 4, 8, 66, 77, 84
Anatomical structures superposition 66
Anatomy 1, 2, 3, 4, 5, 6, 7, 8, 9, 10, 11, 12, 13,
    14, 15, 16, 17, 18, 19, 20, 21, 22, 23, 24,
    25, 26, 27, 28, 29, 30, 31, 32, 33, 34, 35,
    36, 37, 38, 39, 40, 41, 42, 43, 44, 45, 46,
    47, 48, 49, 50, 51, 52, 53, 54, 56, 57, 58,
    59, 60, 61, 62, 63, 64, 65, 66, 67, 68, 69,
    70, 71, 72, 73, 74, 75, 77, 78, 79, 80, 81,
    82, 83, 84, 85
Anatomy
  complex 1
  dental 13
  dental-maxillo-mandibular 5
Anatomy of Extraoral Techniques 56, 57, 59,
    61, 63, 65, 67, 69, 71, 73, 75
Ancient Greek anatome 13
Anomalies 54, 77, 79, 84
  dental 77
  genetic 84
Anterior Mandibular Region 42, 45, 47
Anterior Maxilla Region 46, 48
Anterior Maxillary Region 43
Anterior palatine foramen 21
Apex 5, 6, 21, 35
Arch, dental 77, 81
Areas

radiolucency 2
radiopacity 3
Arrows 78, 79
Assessment 6, 8
Axial 11, 56, 61, 62
Axis, long 5

## B

Basal layer 45
Bite-wing 6
Bone loss 46, 47
  inter-radicular 49
Bones 1, 9, 41, 44, 56, 84
  compact 44
  condensation 53
  destroyed inter-radicular 49
  mandible 34
  radiopaque trabeculae 21
  sphenoid 63
  spongy 44
  trabecular 44
  zygomatic 30, 64
Bone tissue 5, 6
Bony projections 35
Border, lower 34
Brain frontal lobe 63
Branch, mandible 40

## C

Canine 21, 24, 27
  upper 27
Canine and Premolar Region 27, 28, 36, 37, 38
Canine Region 24, 25, 26
Cementoenamel junction 46
CentralRegion 34, 35
Cephalometric Radiography 9, 57, 58
Cephalostat device 9, 10
Cervical portion 44, 49
Conoid tooth 79
Cortical bone, dense 27

Crowns 5, 6, 7, 13, 80
  separated 80
Cysts, globulemaxillary 24

**D**

Deciduous 77, 84
Deciduous dentition 81
Dens Invaginatus 82
Density 2, 4, 41
  high 3
  low 2
  radiographic 3
Dental Radiographic Images 1, 3
Dental Radiographic Techniques 5, 7, 9, 11,
  13
Dentin 13, 15, 81, 84
Dentine 81
Dentin structure 41
Dentistry 41, 66
Dentition, permanent 77, 81
Dilaceration 81, 82
Dilaceration Premolar 81
Direction, opposite 65
Displacement 9, 11, 50
Distortion 4, 6
  minimal 2
Divergence Molar 82
Division 7

**E**

Edges
  anterior 27
  incisal 82
  lower 22
Enamel 3, 13, 81, 84
Enamel hypoplasia 84
Enamel organ cells 82
Enamel radiopacity 13
Enamel structure 84
Ennis 27, 28
Eruption tooth 44
Evaginations 82
Evaluation 8, 9, 10, 77

periodontal 6
prosthetic 7
Examination 9, 66
  clinical 1, 77
  low-cost 5
  radiographic 1, 50
Extraoral Techniques 5, 56, 57, 59, 61, 63, 65,
67, 69, 71, 73, 75

**F**

Facial bones 1
Facial bones subject 64
Facial type 63, 64
Featured Cement 16, 17
Featured Dentin 14, 15
Featured Enamel 14
Featured Floor 22
Featured Intermaxillary suture 23
Featured Pulp Cavity 15, 16
Fibers, oblique 44
Film
  dental 5
  electronic 54
Floor 21, 27, 63
  shallow arch mouth 66
Form anomalies 80
Fractures 9, 11, 27, 63, 64
  mandible 8
Frontal bone forms 63
Frontal View of Skull 64, 66
Frontozygomatic suture 10
Function 1, 41, 44
Furcation 49
Furcation involvement 49, 50
Furcation lesion 49
Furcation size 49
Fusion 80, 81
  differentiated 81

**G**

Gemination 80, 81
Generalized microdontia 79
  relative 79

Gingiva 44, 45
  attached 44
Gingival margin 44
GINGIVAL SULCUS 45
Gingiva recession 49
Gray 2, 3
Grooves 82, 84

**H**

Head 9, 77
Health 1, 5, 6
Hirtz Projection 11, 61, 62
Horizontal Bone Loss 45, 46, 47
Horizontal component, increased 49
Human head dimensions 9
Hutchinson's Tooth 84

**I**

IDEAL RADIOGRAPH 2
Image formation 4
Image layer 65
Images 1, 2, 3, 5, 6, 11, 56, 64, 66
  ideal radiographic 2
  intraoral 66
  radiopacity 30
  sharp radiographic 5
  single 65
  sinus 27
Imperfect amelogenesis 84
Imperfect dentinogenesis 84
Incidence, ray 11
Incisal surfaces 5, 6
Incisive foramen 21
  featured 21
Incisors 82, 84
  central 21, 35
  lower 53
  permanent maxillary 80
  upper 21
Individuals, edentulous 27, 36
Inferior incisor periapical radiography 15, 16,
  18

Inferior molar periapical radiography 14, 15,
  17, 19, 20
Inferior orbital base 63
Inferior View of Skull 59, 60
Inflammation, gingival 46
INTERMAXILLARY SUTURE 22
Interproximal 5, 13, 32, 33
INTERPROXIMAL RADIOGRAPHS 13
Interproximal radiographs record 6
Interproximal Radiography 6
Intersection 27
Intra-oral examinations 66
INTRAORAL EXAMINATIONS 5
Intra-oral radiographs 66
Intraoral Techniques 5, 13, 15, 17, 19, 21, 23,
  25, 27, 29, 31, 33, 35, 37, 39, 41, 43, 45,
  47, 49, 51, 53, 54
Intraoral X-ray equipment 77
Invade 63, 64

**J**

Jaw heads 11
Jaws 44, 56, 79
Jaws fractures 50

**L**

Lamina dura 19, 21, 44
Lateral incisor 21, 24, 27, 82
Lateral Incisor and Canine Region 24, 25, 26
Lateral View of Skull 65
Lesion 49, 77
  pathological 77
  periapical 21
  periodontal 45

**M**

Magnetic resonance imaging (MRI) 9
Mandible Dental Regions 34
Mandibular Occlusal Technique 53, 54
Maxilla 7, 21, 22, 30, 31, 32, 41, 50
  posterior 31

Maxillary Occlusal Technique 50, 51
Maxillary sinus 21, 25, 26, 27, 63, 64
Maxillary sinus extensions 27
Maxillary sinus floor 27
Maxillary sinus region 8
Maxillary Tuberosity 27, 34
Maxillomandibular 13, 66
Maxillo-mandibular 5, 13, 56, 77
Mental foramen 36
Mental spine 35
Mental spines protrude 53
Microdontia 79, 80
   unidental 79
Middle 40, 56, 63
Middle fossa 63
Middle portion 40
Middle region 63
Midline 21, 35
Modern diagnostic image 1
Molar Region 27, 28, 29, 30, 31, 32, 33, 38,
       39, 40
Molar region toothless 29
Molars 27, 36, 40, 84
   mulberry 84
   upper 30
Morphological alterations 9
Morphological characteristics, normal 80
Morphology, craniofacial 1
Mouth 66, 72, 73, 74, 75
   open 64
Mouth exam 6, 7
Mouth intraoral radiographs 8
MRI (magnetic resonance imaging) 9

**N**

Nasal cavity 10, 21, 27, 63
   featured 22
Nasal fossa 21, 22, 27
Neurocranium 56
Normal anatomical structure 13, 56, 66, 77
Normal Periodontium 42, 43
Nostrils 22
Nutrition 41, 44

**O**

Object 2, 6
   radiographed 2, 3
Object densities 3
Object distortion 6
Oblique orbital lines 63
Occipital-frontal direction 10
Occlusal 5, 6
Occlusal films 50
Occlusal plane 36
Occlusal radiographs 27, 50
Occlusal radiography 7, 8, 50
Occlusal surfaces 7
Occlusal trauma 47, 49
Oral cavity 5, 8, 65
Orbits 10
Overlapping shadow 22

**P**

PA (Posterior Anterior) 59, 67, 68
Palatines 27, 34, 56
Panoramic Radiograph 5, 65, 69, 70, 71, 72
Panoramic radiography 8, 56, 77
Panoramic radiography. *See* PR
Panoramic radiography equipment 9
PA Projection 10, 11, 63
PA Skull 10
Pathologies 1, 10, 54, 56, 77, 79, 81, 83, 84,
       85
Patient 8, 54, 56, 65, 77
   edentulous 63, 64
Patient anatomy 66
Patient characteristics 1
Patient motion 66
Patient position 66
Patient positioning 9
Patient's condition 1
PA Waters 63, 64
Periapical Radiographs 5, 6, 21, 22, 23, 24, 25,
       26, 27, 28, 29, 30, 31, 32, 34, 35, 36, 37,
       38, 39, 40, 41, 42, 43, 45, 46, 47, 48, 49,
       50, 53
Periapical Radiography 5

Periodontal disease 44, 45, 49
Periodontal ligament 16, 17, 41, 44, 45
Periodontitis 49
Periodontium 41
Periodontium Regions 41
Positioners 6
Posteiror Mandibular Region 42
Posterior Anterior (PA) 59, 67, 68
Posterior Mandibular Region 46, 48
Posterior Maxilla Region 43, 47, 49
PR (Panoramic radiography) 8, 9, 56, 65, 66, 77
Premolar and Molar Region 27, 28, 29, 33
Premolar Region 27, 28, 32, 34, 36, 37, 38
Premolars 36, 79
Pres molar and molar 27
Probing 45
Probing depth 44
Projection, correct radiographic 1
Projection technique 10
Protection Periodontium 41, 44
Pulp chamber 80, 81, 82

**R**

Radiation beam, narrow 65
Radiation dose reduction 8
Radiographic 45
Radiographic appearance 44
Radiographic cephalometry 9
Radiographic contrast 3
Radiographic films 4, 5, 6, 7
Radiographic film/sensor parallel 7
Radiographic findings 1
Radiographic image 2, 3, 4, 13, 21, 30, 36, 56, 65, 77, 81
Radiographic interpretation 1
Radiographic quality 4
Radiographic shots 9
Radiographs 1, 6, 31, 45, 77
Radiography 1, 2, 3, 49
  dental 1
  extraoral 5
  intraoral 5, 8
Radiolucent area 27, 35

Radiolucent images 14, 21, 46
  oval 21
  rounded 36
Radiolucent lines 21, 22, 36
  oblique 64
  thick 36
Radiolucent line skirting, thin 20
Radiopaque 13, 19, 30, 35, 44
Radiopaque edge 36
Radiopaque image 13, 31, 32, 34
  well-defined 13
Radiopaque lines 21, 25, 26, 27, 34, 40, 41, 44
  thick 21
Radiopaque region 22
Radiopaque structure 21
Reduction 46
Region 4, 5, 7, 21, 30, 77
  anterior 64
  apical 36
  basilar 56
  cingulate 82
  dental 7, 13
  elongated radiolucent 24
  incisor 34
  neck 9, 77
  posterior 21
  superior central 21
Request 77
Roots 7, 36, 49, 80, 81, 82
  conical 84
  dental 20
  molar 40
  natural morphology 49
  residual 50

**S**

Sensor 5, 6
Sensor head 65
Sensor positioning devices 54
Sensory effect 41
Sensory organs 56
Shades 2, 3
Shadows, radiographic 13
Sinuses, maxillary 9, 10, 11, 63

SINUS MAXILLARY 27
Skull 1, 11, 56, 59, 60, 61, 64, 65, 66
Skull Radiograph 59
Sockets 44
  dental 44
Soft tissue retraction 49
Soft tissues 1, 2, 9, 49
  evaluating 50
Spaces 20, 63, 64
  interradicular 49
  radiolucent marrow 21
Sphenoid 56
Sphenoid foramen ovale 63
Sphenoid sinus 11, 64
Structures 1, 5, 11, 13, 65, 77, 84
  dental 5
  facial 65
  metal 3
  multiple superimposed 1
  neighboring 5
  normal 13
  overlapping 7
  support 5
  surrounding 8, 54
  trabecular 44
Superior and inferior incisor periapical
      radiography 15, 16
Superior and inferior molar periapical
      radiography 14, 15, 17
Superior incisor periapical radiography 17, 19,
      21, 22, 23
Superior Incisor Region 23, 24
Superior molar periapical radiography 18, 20
Supernumerary roots 83
Supernumerary teeth 77, 78
Support periodontium 41

T

Taurodontism 82, 83
Techniques 1, 5, 6, 7, 10, 11, 12, 65
  bisector 5
  extraoral radiographic 5
  interproximal 5, 6
  radiographic 5, 11

Teeth 5, 6, 7, 13, 19, 63, 64, 77, 79, 81, 83
  anterior 81
  extracted 64
  impacted 50
  lower 7
  missing 63
  molar 27
  multirooted 49
  permanent 84
  two 80
Teeth fixation 41
Teeth germ 80
Teleradiograph 9, 10
Temporomandibular dysfunction 9
Temporomandibular Joint Radiograph 72, 73,
      74, 75
Temporomandibular Joint Radiography 9
Tissue fluid 44
Tissues 41
  calcified 84
  connective 44, 45
  dense modeled conjunctive 44
  dental 54
  dentinal 84
  hard tooth 13
  keratinized 45
  periodontal 20, 45
  resistant 44
TMJ (Temporalmandibular Joint) 9, 56, 65, 67
TMJ radiography 9
Tones 3
Tooth 5, 14, 21, 44, 45, 49, 79, 80
  adjacent 81
  deciduous 84
  gemination 80
  posterior 82
Tooth apex 14
Tooth development 8
Tooth mobility 44
Tooth relation 6
Tooth root 44
Tooth sockets 44
Trauma 9, 10, 81, 84
  direct 64
  multiple 22
  occlusion 47

surgical 64
Trauma acts 47
Traumatic 77
Tuberosity 27, 34
Turner's tooth 84

## U

Union 34, 81
    cementum 44
Upper Canine Occlusal 52

## V

Variations 3, 13, 44, 82
    anatomical 77
Vertical Bone Loss 45, 47, 48, 49
Viscerocranium 56

## W

Waters projection 10
Water's technique 63
Wing 63

## X

X-ray source 65

## Z

Zygomatic 56, 64
Zygomatic arch 11
Zygomatic extension 27
Zygomatic Process 30
Zygomatic-temporal suture 64

www.ingramcontent.com/pod-product-compliance
Lightning Source LLC
Chambersburg PA
CBHW041720210326
41598CB00007B/727